Table of Conte

MW00907879

Alternate Titles Considered:

(FYI- I went with the more positive title-other titles considered for this book)-
Deadly Advice! Deadly Neglect, How Mainstream Medicine Makes & Keeps
You Sick to Keep the Profits $$ Rolling In! The Conspiracy Uncovered
OR
Never Get Sick Again! Cancel Your Health Insurance! Then Fire Your Doctor!
Correct The 5 Deadly Deficiencies of The Modern Age and Easily Take Back
Your Health & All Your $Money$ From the $Medical Mafia$)

What is Modern Medicine?

My father, a Stanford-educated MD and surgeon, inadvertently summed it up one day in one sentence. He explained to me "Jeff, every medicine in reality is actually a poison". That seemed a bit shocking to me at first, but I now know what he was trying to say. For ages, modern medicine has basically been a replacement for your normally functioning immune system that kills off bad actors like viruses, bacteria, fungi, and cancer cells. When your immune system for some reason is not doing its job, doctors step in and try to fashion a man-made replacement for the segment of your immune system that is not working.

4

So, your body won't kill off that infection by itself? No problem, go get an antibiotic -that should do the trick. The antibiotic is a poison that will kill off the bacteria in the infection that is very poisonous to bacteria and much less poisonous to you.

The problem is, your body should have prevented or handled the infection in the first place; if you did get an infection your immune system should have quickly killed it off. The doctors aren't treating the true problem; **the true problem is that there is something wrong with your immune system.** Modern medicine is just acting as a surrogate immune system that comes into play when yours is not working properly. Doctors have poisons for all sorts of diseases, or they will resort to surgery if the poisons don't work (a true admission of failure) but they never attack the real problem- fixing your immune system so that you never get sick in the first place. Fixing your immune system so that you never get sick again is what you will learn how to do in this book.

Now lately, modern medicine has been making steps in the right direction. They have finally started trying to fix your immune system so that it does its job. This can be seen in the rise of the "biologics" that are drugs designed **to rev up** one small part of your immune system to attack a certain disease like cancer or infections, **or oppositely** to **suppress** one small segment of your immune system that accidentally attacks good tissues which causes autoimmune diseases like MS, lupus, psoriasis, etc. If you pay attention to the huge number of ads on tv touting these drugs you will see a pattern:

Every biologic that revs up your immune system to attack bad actors like infecting bacteria, viruses, or fungi, or spontaneously emergent cancer cells (yes, our bodies generate cancer cells every day), almost **all have side effects that include the triggering of various autoimmune diseases.**

The revved-up part of the immune system often kills off the cancer cells or infection but then goes into overdrive at times and starts attacking your good tissues. Thus**, the side effects of cancer biologics almost always include the triggering of autoimmune diseases.**

Here is a list of the possible side effects of Keytruda used to treat the skin cancer melanoma, it reads like a who's who of tissues attacked in autoimmune diseases>>

SIDE EFFECTS

- Immune-mediated pneumonitis. (lungs)
- Immune-mediated colitis (intestines)
- Immune-mediated hepatitis and hepatotoxicity (liver)

- Immune-mediated endocrinopathies (adrenal/hormonal glands)
- Immune-mediated nephritis and renal dysfunction (kidneys)
- Immune-mediated skin adverse reactions
- Other immune-mediated adverse reactions
- Infusion-related reactions

Likewise, when you see an ad for a biologic for autoimmune diseases that suppresses part of the immune system to stop it from attacking your good tissues, the side effects are almost always infections and cancers!

Here are some of the side effects listed for the best-selling biologic Humira which is used to treat various autoimmune disorders such as Crohn's disease and plaque psoriasis. By shutting down part of your immune system attack, it inadvertently allows bad actors like cancer cells and infecting organisms to slip by. **So, the side effects of autoimmune biologics are almost always cancers and infections.**

"A black box warning in Humira's label highlights the risk of serious infections leading to hospitalization or death, including TB, bacterial sepsis, invasive fungal infections and **infections** due to opportunistic pathogens. It also features **cancers,** notably lymphoma and hepatosplenic T-cell lymphoma. "

What will be revealed to you shortly in this book is the identity of the ultimate biologic-

that **revs up** the attacking part of your immune system to attack bad actors, while simultaneously **tamping down** the part of your immune system that attacks good tissues. With NO SIDE EFFECTS!

This substance is cheap, unpatentable, easily available, and eventually will put many drug companies and doctors out of business after its widespread adoption by the general public.

Now let's look at another function of your body that sometimes goes haywire and causes chronic conditions- let's look at your tissue remodeling system.

What is your tissue remodeling system? It is that function of your body that is in charge of repairing injuries, breaking down and rebuilding incorrect tissue types like cysts, bone spurs, bunions, etc. It is even in charge of continually breaking down and rebuilding normal bones and tissues just to keep them fresh and new! When the tissue remodeling system is malfunctioning, the doctors have another simple solution- get out a scalpel and do the remodeling work for you! This highlights the other part of modern medicine's tool kit-   surgery.

Surgery seems sophisticated at first glance, but it is actually where doctors perform functions in your body that are supposed to be done by your remodeling system but are not.

Rather than fixing your remodeling system to rebuild your body according to the blueprints in the DNA in every cell in your body, the surgeons just go in and cut and slash to do what your faulty remodeling system is supposed to be doing. Many, and perhaps almost the vast majority of surgeries can be avoided by simply getting your remodeling system to start operating properly! Pardon the pun.

 (I of course exclude surgery required to repair severe injuries from the category of unnecessary. Severe injuries are one area where we will always need skilled surgeons).

Now this is what you might find truly unbelievable-the substance that will perfectly tune up your immune system to prevent and cure virtually every disease known is <u>also</u> the master conductor of your <u>tissue-remodeling</u> system! They are two sides of the same coin! The ultimate biologic described earlier is also your ultimate tissue remodeling hormone!

And the great thing about this magical immune system and tissue remodeling hormone is that it is completely non-toxic at virtually any dose as long as you understand it and use it carefully with a few conditions which I will share with you later.

Most doctors will tell you this substance is very dangerous at low doses and you should never take it at the doses high enough to restore your heath and prevent all illness and chronic conditions! They will yell at you and tell you these doses are dangerous and toxic! They are so, so wrong- and we will have to ask later, do they really want to be right? Because if there is an actual substance that will fine tune your immune and remodeling systems- the need for doctors, hospitals, and Big Pharma will plunge by at least 90%! Your own body will perform most medical diagnoses, procedures and cures, the way it was originally designed, as opposed to your doctor trying to serve as a vastly inferior replacement for your body's immune and self-repair functions.

And this substance is just one of five that you need to take to be able to fire your doctor, cancel your health insurance and never get sick again.

Are you skeptical? Of course you are, and you should be! But soon enough I expect to change your mind-so let's get started.

Introduction:

I am shortly going to tell you something right now that is going to seem unbelievable!

And unless you are a completely naïve, you are going to throw up your hands, and laugh-IMPOSSIBLE! And rightly so- it will be an outrageous claim that is so extraordinary that the only way anyone could ever believe it is if they are confronted with extraordinary proof-which often is usually an insurmountable standard. But this book will provide that extraordinary proof -in your face and undeniable-just wait and see. There will be MOUNTAINS of extraordinary proof to consider!

And if I had not spent the many years looking into many thousands of studies, and hearing from thousands of people about their illnesses and their months' and years' long self-experiments to cure themselves, I too would laugh and say IMPOSSIBLE! And maybe smugly toss this book into the garbage can.

Your next reason for not reading any further would be the question who is this

Jeff T. Bowles and what could he possibly know?

If you haven't read my bestselling book about this ultimate biologic (which has sold 300,000+ copies and has been translated into 10 languages) then let me give you a few tidbits for now. In 2011, I conducted an experiment on myself and got dramatic results with this ultimate biologic. Chronic issues and diseases I had had for 20+ years disappeared after a few months to a few years (two years for a 100% cure of seasonal allergies- 90%improvement after one year). Decades old allergies, cysts, bone spurs, arthritic shoulders, near sightedness, were all just miraculously cured after I boosted my daily dosage of this ultimate biologic to what doctors called "dangerous levels". At the same time of my self- experimentation, I also read/studied every abstract in the PubMed medical database concerning this ultimate biologic during that year. There were 54,000 of them at that time around 2010-2011. I have read thousands more since then. And since then I have heard from more than 1,000 people conducting high dose experiments on themselves and they are finding cures for everything from MS to lupus to psoriasis to chronic infections, etc. etc. which I have added to a big search engine. Can this ultimate biologic cure your disease? More on this soon.

Also, I come from a long line of Stanford educated doctors – a grandfather, father and 2 uncles; medical research is in my blood and I just can't stop! Not a surprise that I grew up in complete awe of and with great admiration for modern medicine, so I do not take writing this book lightly, and it took almost a lifetime of evidence to finally convince me of the shocking truth about modern medicine.

In 1998 and 2000 I published 3 theory papers regarding aging and disease which were accelerated for publication because the editors said the papers were extremely exciting and of major importance. The editorial board of the journal has had editors that shared five Nobel prizes amongst them (as of the year 1998) and several had been knighted by the Queen of England for their discoveries. Based on my test score for the graduate school admissions test I have a Mensa-level IQ (having a high IQ, I believe, just makes it relatively easier for a person to recognize patterns in obscure sets of data). So enough about me. How about you?

What do you have to lose by reading this book? Maybe a couple of hours? Not a big gamble. What could you stand to gain? How about tens if not hundreds of thousands of dollars saved over a lifetime in health insurance premiums and out of pocket medical costs, not to mention a lifetime of good health with virtually no diseases or medical issues at least until you get past the age of 50 or so (Don't worry I've got something for aging too which was the original area of my life long research). And think of your family and children as well! Skipping childhood cancers, asthma, eczema, and autism would be nice too right? So even if there is only a 1% chance that what I am going to tell you is true, it would still be foolish for you not to read this book from cover to cover.

After I make the seemingly outrageous claims below, I will then provide you with the extraordinary proof you will need to realize that what I say is true!

Okay are you ready? Here we go-

Virtually all diseases we face in the modern era that are not caused by post-age 50 aging or genetic mutations are caused by five widespread deficiencies.

I call them the five deadly deficiencies of the modern age. The first one below is what I have been calling the ultimate biologic. It is now revealed to you as Vitamin D3-not a vitamin at all but a powerful immune system and remodeling system controlling hormone. The other 4 deficiencies that plague the modern age and cause most other illnesses and chronic conditions are Magnesium, Vitamin K2, boron and zinc deficiencies. (Boron and zinc are bit players on this list at this time, but boron has been shown to cure arthritis in some people, and zinc has been shown to regrow your thymus and rejuvenate your immune system).

THE 5 DEADLY DEFCIECNIES OF THE
MODERN AGE-

Vitamin D3 Deficiency (The ultimate biologic &
tissue remodeler)
Magnesium Deficiency (A missing dietary element
that causes many diseases)
Vitamin K2 Deficiency (Vitamin D3's important
helper)
Boron Deficiency (A builder of strong bones and
joints)
Zinc Deficiency (A powerful immune system
builder)

Now keep in mind that many of the diseases
associated with each deficiency may overlap into
the other deficiency categories, for example heart
disease is associated with three of the above
deficiencies, while migraine headaches are
associated with both Vitamin D3 and magnesium
deficiencies. Prostate cancer is associated with D3
and K2 deficiencies while arthritis is associated
with boron, K2, and D3 deficiencies. Maybe we
will ultimately find out they are all connected to all
the diseases we face, but for now these are some of
the obvious interacting deficiencies.

The fact that there are a lot of interactions between
these deficiencies has clouded the research waters

for decades as scientists typically look for and investigate single variables to find cures for various diseases.

Only by working with and understanding multiple variables simultaneously can we reveal the cause of almost all diseases of the modern age.

("Unbelievable!" do I hear you say?)

STOP! DO NOT THROW THIS BOOK IN THE TRASH!

I will now give you a brief summary of how this is possible and is true! Bear with me just one more page.

What is this Magical Vitamin D3?

The most important deficiency that causes maybe 75% of all disease is Vitamin D3 deficiency. Not only does Vitamin D3 deficiency cause 75% of all disease, high doses of Vitamin D3 can cure up to 75% of all diseases- more on this later.

Vitamin D3 IS NOT A VITAMIN!

It doesn't even fit the definition of a vitamin!

Vitamin-noun

1. Any of a group of organic compounds which are essential for normal growth and nutrition and are required in small quantities in the diet **because they cannot be synthesized by the body.**

You **can** make Vitamin D3 in your body from cholesterol by just sitting in the sun and letting the sun hit your skin!

What is Vitamin D3? It is actually a steroid hormone that controls or affects at least 2,700+ genes by my count and likely many more. Most of these genes are involved in immune system regulation and tissue remodeling. More on this shortly.

(Note: in order to try and get the price of this paperback down to $9.99 instead of $13.99- I had

17

to minimize or eliminate many pictures and illustrations. I have also omitted most of the appendices. But don't worry! You can just send me an email at -

BannedCovidBook@gmail.com

and I will send you a pdf file with everything that was removed. Don't worry the things that were removed were just some extra fun bells and whistles and do not detract from the value and information content of this book.)

VITAMIN D3

Why was it named Vitamin D3? Because it was first discovered that dogs kept indoors remained healthy if they consumed Vitamin D in their diet, and when it was withheld, they developed deformed legs due to the disease called rickets This is the first example of a tissue (bone) remodeling disease that researchers learned was caused by Vitamin D deficiency.

18

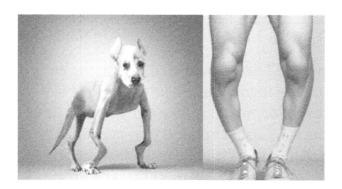

Dog with Rickets/**Humans can get rickets too, but in older days it used to be called being bow-legged.**

They later realized when the dogs were raised in sunlight that they did not need Vitamin D in their diet to prevent rickets, thus it was realized Vitamin D was not a vitamin. Yet to this day it is still called Vitamin D simply because it was discovered after Vitamin C! It's that simple and that stupid.

So how did so many of us become Vitamin D3 deficient? It's a long story but in summary, doctors since the 1930's have been mistakenly taught that "high doses" (which aren't really high) of Vitamin D2 and D3 are dangerous, and since the 1980's, due to doctors' skin cancer scares, most Americans have been avoiding the sun and using sunscreen which prevents Vitamin D3 production in the skin. Low oral Vitamin D intake combined with large scale sun avoidance/sunscreen use **has led to a**

19

rampant epidemic of a huge number of diseases and chronic conditions since the 1980's. More on this shortly. Let's backtrack for a moment.

Vitamin D2 was discovered first in the early 1900's when they found that when you shined UV light on some organic material like mushrooms that the mushrooms could be used to prevent rickets. It turns out that UV light caused the mushrooms to make Vitamin D2. Vitamin D2 is the plant-based version of the hormone that is slightly different in chemical structure from the animal version which is Vitamin D3. Vitamin D2 mostly has the same effects of Vitamin D3 but it is about $1/4^{th}$ to $1/16^{th}$ as active in humans as D3-and it is much more likely to have negative side effects at truly high doses as compared to Vitamin D3. Interestingly, the chemical name for Vitamin D2 is ergocalciferol-the "ergot" is Latin for fungus/mushroom. Vitamin D3 is called cholecalciferol from the Latin root of chole- for bile. In the 1930's it was found that if one prevented the production of bile in the rat that Vitamin D3 could not be absorbed. Also, around this time Vitamin D3 was discovered as a component in cod liver oil that prevented dogs raised indoors from getting rickets.

In the 1920's -

The public started taking both Vitamin D2 and D3 in droves, along with many other recently discovered vitamins.

One version of the early Vitamin D story as noted by encyclopedia.com goes like this…

"During the 1920's vitamin craze that followed Funk's discoveries, many people overlooked Funk's observation that only small amounts of the substances were necessary to maintain health. Nutritional supplements were said to cure diseases, and vitamin makers claimed that synthetic vitamins improved energy and health. **Consumers began to ingest large amounts of vitamins**, despite the fact that small amounts were sufficient and that **too much of some vitamins, such as Vitamin A & D are toxic to the body."**

Now there is **another version of the story** that I heard which originated from a respected medical professor at Canada's McGill university, and before I share it with you, consider this-

In the late 1800's, around the US, there was a boom in hospital construction that continued into the 1900's and was going strong in 1910. In the U.S., the number of hospitals reached 4400 in 1910, and they provided 420,000 beds while the US population was only 92 million (**1 bed for every 220 people**). The 1920 Census showed 6,613 registered hospitals in the US a 50% increase over 1910!

Compare this to the number of hospitals in 2016 in the US: 6,200 hospitals with 890,000 beds for a population of 323 million people. (**1 bed for every 363 people**)

By all measures the US had an overabundance of hospitals relative to the population in the 1910s and even more so by the 1920s.

Hospital Capacity and General Population, 1872-1932

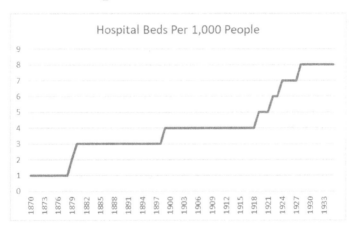

Hospital Beds Per 1,000 People

Data Source: "Hospital Service in the United States: Twelfth Annual Presentation of Hospital Data by the Council on Medical Education and Hospitals of the American Medical Association," *JAMA 100*, 12(March 25, 1933)

Hospital Beds per 1,000 people in 2019: 2.4!

By the 1920s, the hospital was a place where people expected that illness might be treated and even cured. In the roaring 20's not-for-profit hospitals began reducing their traditional charitable role in favor of creating prestigious institutions attractive to a well-paying upper middle class. Between 1865 and 1925 in all regions of the United States, hospitals transformed into expensive, modern hospitals of science and technology. They served increasing numbers of paying middle-class patients. **In the process, they experienced increased financial pressures and competition**. Between 1909 and 1932, the number of hospital beds increased six times as fast as the general population, leading experts to assert in 1933 that **the country was "over-hospitalized".**

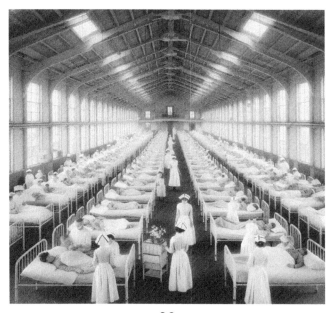

Now here is the alternate version of the history of the vitamin craze of the 1920's:

According to one scientist's account, the average person in the late 1920's and early 1930's was taking 20 to 25mg of Vitamin D2 or D3 per day, **and soon the hospitals were virtually empty-nobody was getting sick anymore.** The hospitals were all about to go bankrupt along with the doctors and drug companies. (*Quote attributed to the late famous Vitamin D/Calcium Researcher Dr. Carl Reich in Robert Barefoot's book "The Disease Conspiracy-The FDA Suppression of Cures" 2006 page 141.*)

Vitamin D became available to the general public. It was touted as the Sunshine Vitamin and soon there was a Vitamin D craze. Food manufacturers were putting Vitamin D in everything from hot dogs to beer. Often food producers could just shine UV light on various foodstuffs to increase their Vitamin D content.

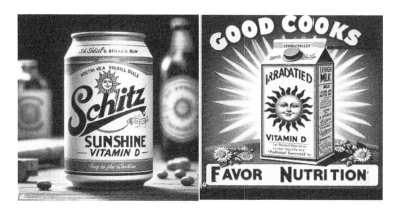

From 1928

So How Did Mainstream Medicine Respond to The Miracle of The Sunshine Hormone Vitamin D Causing the Hospitals to Become Empty?

Their first action was to change the unit of measurement of Vitamin D from milligrams to International Units which we use today. **<u>All of the sudden 25 mg became 1 million International Units- which sounds much scarier indeed!</u>**

Also, a study was performed where 7 medical students were convinced to take massive enough doses of Vitamin D (likely impure) to kill a horse (in the long run), and lo and behold the students got very sick, the experiment was stopped and they recovered.   That was all that was needed, and medical authorities pressured Vitamin D manufacturers and retailers to take Vitamin D off the market.

As expected, there was a public outcry and the government in 1928 decided to commission a comprehensive study of the question of Vitamin D toxicity with the University of Illinois at Chicago. The study lasted 9 years, involved hundreds of doctors and 773 humans and 63 dogs, and resulted in what is known as the Steck report (but often mistakenly called the Streck report on the internet). This report basically concluded that doses up to 20,000 IU per kilogram of body weight per day (or 1 million IU's per the typical woman of 50 kgs/110 pounds) were safely tolerated in dogs for indeterminate lengths of time even when taken for years. **The report blamed prior cases of toxicity on improper production techniques and stated that the new "Whittier" process eliminated Vitamin D toxicity**.

Amongst the humans, who were given doses of up to 200,000 IU a day for periods of seven days to five years there were no deaths. And one of the authors of the report took 3 million IU's a day for 15 days without any evidence of disturbance of any kind. And finally, they found "Vitamin D intoxication" by taking much higher amounts of Vitamin D for short periods did not result in any recognizable permanent injury. The final conclusion was that the burden of proof had shifted to those who maintained the undesirability of high dose Vitamin D therapy.

Well, the findings in the Steck report were ignored by mainstream medicine, and **since the early 1930's people were warned not to take any more than 400 IUs of Vitamin D** per day because it might be toxic!

More than 400 IU being dangerous is especially ridiculous when you consider that whole body sunbathing for just thirty minutes produces 20,000 IU of Vitamin D3 in your skin! And since the 1930's 400 IU's per day of Vitamin D3 has been the recommended amount of Vitamin D we are all supposed to take according to doctors and the drug industry-barely enough to keep infants from getting rickets and our bones becoming soft!

This is an OUTRAGEOUS scandal!

Oh yeah, and what happened to the huge number of hospitals, doctors, and the drug companies all about to go bankrupt in the early 1930's? They were all saved. As soon as the population stopped taking "dangerous" doses of Vitamin D the hospitals quickly filled up again and have remained full ever since.

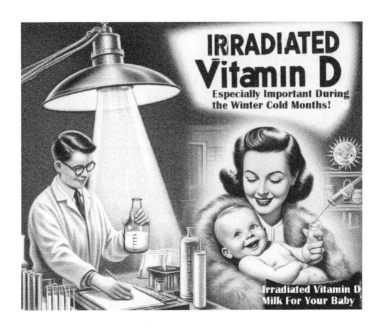

So, scientists and drug companies were telling us in the 1930's that any amount of Vitamin D over 400 IU's may be toxic! But somehow the drug industry saw fit to create three new miracle drugs for use in treating cancer and other diseases with the brand names Dalsol, Deltalin, and Drisdol. Each of these drugs was nothing more than a daily pill containing 50,000 IU of Vitamin D2 or D3 and a filler. The drug industry was not doing well during the depression years of the 1930's and these "new" drugs that actually worked saved them financially, all the while they were telling the public anything over 400 IUs per day was toxic. (I have a few modern case reports of people curing late stage cancer with 50,000 IU of D3 per day in the chapter on cancer coming up).

Since the 1930's there has been a long unbroken chain of hostility from the medical community and the FDA against Vitamin D supplements that continues to this day. Bill after bill, law after law, have been proposed over the years to prevent Vitamin D fortification of foods, to prevent the sale of higher dose Vitamin D3 pills, and to reclassify vitamins as drugs!

From my 2014 nexus article…

The campaign started in New York in 1944 when the attorney general Nathaniel Goldstein ruled that vitamins were drugs and could only be sold by pharmacists and registered drug stores. This ruling was quickly challenged in court and overturned. But Big Pharma was not going to just give up easily.

In 1952 the FDA (Food & Drug Association) tried to outlaw the introduction of anything "new" into foods and consumables unless given advanced affirmative permission by the FDA. This power grab was rejected by the courts. In 1957 the FDA started prosecution of vendors of "malnutrition remedies" (AKA vitamins) and began using the term "quack".

In 1960 the FDA tried to limit the amount of folic acid in vitamins to .4 of a milligram even though years later this amount would be found to be too low and higher amounts were recommended for pregnant mothers to prevent neural tube defects in their newborns.

In 1966 again the FDA tried to restrict access to vitamins by the food industry by proposing new controls on Vitamin D fortification.

In 1973 the FDA banned the sale of higher dose Vitamin A and Vitamin D pills. This was later challenged by Linus Pauling, the Nobel Prize winning chemist, as a friend of the court in a lawsuit against the FDA.

In 1974 Congress reigned in the FDA's overreach and forced them to regulate vitamins as food and not drugs.

In 1976 Congress also passed a bill blocking the FDA and the drug industry's attempts to block the sale of high dose vitamins.

In 1977 the FDA dropped its plans to require a doctor's prescription for high dose vitamins.

But in 1979, the FDA tried again to get some vitamins classified as non-prescription drugs…another small first step towards later banning.

1992: The FDA with Texas state health inspectors raided vitamin retailers/ health food stores across the state and seized inventories and put people in jail accusing the businessmen of making false health claims about vitamins.

1993: FDA planned to regulate vitamins again and health claims about them.

Finally: in 1994 the people of the US had had enough and they forced Congress to pass the US Dietary Supplement Health and Education Act (DSHEA) which is basically "health-freedom" legislation. DSHEA defines supplements as foods, and puts the onus on the United States Food and Drug Administration (FDA) to prove that a supplement poses significant or unreasonable risk of harm rather than on the manufacturer to prove the supplement's safety, reversing the burden of evidence required of medicines. They never quit though.

In 2011 some corrupt, bought and paid for, nanny-statist US politicians tried a back door maneuver to regain control over vitamins and supplements by the FDA with their introduction of the Dietary Supplement Labeling Act of 2011.

Their intent was to overthrow the effect of the 1994 DSHEA law which led to consumers having wide access to dietary supplements. They wanted to change what was essentially a notification

<u>process into a costly approval process</u>. The net effect of the proposed regulation was to reclassify many nutritional compounds currently on the market as new dietary ingredients requiring FDA approval. Luckily for the US population this recent backdoor power grab attempt also failed. But you can bet the corrupted, nanny-state politicians owned by Big Pharma will be at it again sooner or later.

The current attempt to outlaw Vitamin D3 is occurring in Europe where they are debating and trying to get all countries to agree on a single overarching law called the **Codex Alimentarius,** or "Food Code" which is a collection of standards, guidelines and codes of practice adopted by the **Codex Alimentarius** Commission. Once this Food Code is agreed upon by all countries it becomes the law of the land for the participants which includes the US. One thing they are trying to do here is -you guessed it- outlaw high dose Vitamin D3. A recent proposal was that Vitamin D3 daily requirements per person should be 200 to 600 IU's per day! There was a dissenting opinion suggesting it should be   800 to 1000 IU's! BOTH estimates are criminally low!

As you can clearly see, if it were up to Big Pharma, the FDA, paid for congressmen, and many doctors, Vitamin D3 would be a controlled substance available by prescription only, and only in very small doses! Whatever happened to "do no harm"?

A little more interesting history of Vitamin D before we move onto the overwhelming proof section. Sorry, I can't help it, I find it so interesting!

The first Vitamin D pill to obtain the approval of the American Medical Association was Oscodal, a sugar-coated tablet of Vitamin A and D made from cod-liver oil using a process developed by Casimir Funk in the early 1920s. Casimir Funk could be considered the father of the vitamin age as he

discovered a large number of the common vitamins.

In 1923, American biochemist Harry Steenbock at the University of Wisconsin demonstrated that irradiation by ultraviolet light increased the Vitamin D content of foods and other organic materials After irradiating rodent food, Steenbock discovered the rodents were cured of rickets. A Vitamin D deficiency is a known cause of rickets. Steenbock patented his invention. His irradiation technique was used for foodstuffs, most memorably for milk. By the expiration of his patent in 1945, rickets had been all but eliminated in the US.

In 1924 it was found that rats suffering from rickets induced by a low-phosphate diet benefited from irradiation by UV light, not only by irradiation of the rats themselves, but also by irradiation of the "air" in the glass jars from which they had been removed and then put back after irradiation.(It later turned out that it was the irradiated sawdust, feces, and spilled food left in the jars, which the rats later ate, and not the air that improved the rats' rickets.)

Hariette Chick and her co-workers, in 1922, working with malnourished children in a clinic in post-World War I Vienna, showed that rickets prevalent in the children could be cured by whole milk or cod-liver oil.

In the meantime, an entirely different cure for rickets appeared, in the role of UV light. A long-standing tradition held that fresh air and sunshine were good for the prevention of rickets. Hess and Unger, in 1921, put forward the explanation of their clinical observations that "seasonal incidence of rickets is due to seasonal variations of sunlight."

The field received a new impetus when Huldschinsky in 1919 argued that, if sunlight at the seaside or in the mountains can prevent or cure rickets, then artificial sunlight, simulating light at mountain heights should do the same.

He exposed severely rachitic (having rickets) children to irradiation with a quartz-mercury lamp (emitting UV light) every other day for 2 to 20 min for 2 months and observed great improvement, including fresh calcium deposition, as revealed by X-rays. He was careful to make sure that the children had not been exposed to sunlight or received any supplements to their diet during those months.

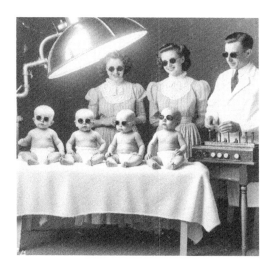

And for many years thereafter, sunlamps were a common household appliance well into the 1960's. It was in the 60's, I remember as a small boy sunbathing with my sister in my parents' bedroom on a blanket on the floor under a mercury vapor lamp. And keep in mind that my father was a Stanford educated MD, so artificial tanning was considered healthy as late as the 1960's and early 1970's. And indeed it was! It caused our skin to produce large amounts of Vitamin D3 even in the middle of the winter! In fact, just ½ hour of UV light exposure can produce around 20,000 IUs of D3 in the skin in the average adult-so these UV lamps were in effect high dose Vitamin D3 therapy! But real healing that PREVENTS and CURES disease <u>cannot be tolerated</u> by the medical community for too long. Sometime by the 1980's these UV lamps had been given the reputation of "quack" medical devices by the medical community and they fell out of favor with the public even though many dermatologists still used UV lamps to treat acne!

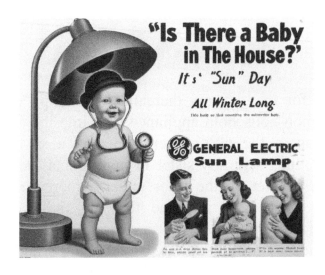

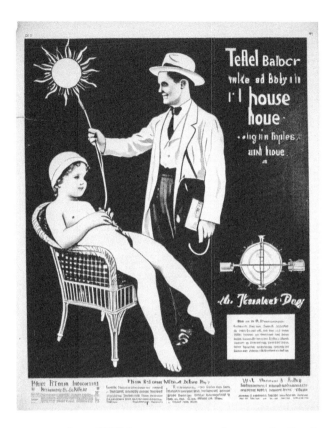

It turns out that UV lamps weren't quack devices at all! By dramatically raising Vitamin D3 levels they were much more effective than most drugs produced by Big Pharma and cures offered by doctors.

These Truly Heath-Boosting Devices of Old are Now Being Labeled and Sold as Medical Curiosities-
 "Quack" Medical Devices / UV-lamps on eBay.>>

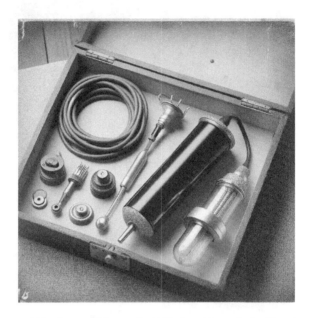

Antique Violetta Electric Violet Ray Medical Device **Quack** Medicine & Box

$29.99

The Overwhelming Proof That Vitamin D3 Deficiency Causes Most Human Diseases-

Introduction-

An interesting question to ask is: why do people have whiter skin the further away from the equator they live (for many generations)?

Answer: Because their darker-skinned ancestors who lived in the same area for some reason died faster than their lighter-skinned ancestors (skin color differences were produced by mutations). So over time, very northern populations became lighter skinned. Why?

Because darker skin takes much longer and stronger sun to make Vitamin D3 than lighter skin. So, by definition as people migrated north from Africa, they all became Vitamin D3 deficient. Away from the strong sun, lighter-skinned mutants tended to survive while darker-skinned migrants perished at much higher rates from Vitamin D3 deficiency diseases.

Lighter-skinned people have become more and more adapted to the weaker sunlight and lower Vitamin D3 levels of the northern climates over time. However, once whiter people recently started avoiding direct sun exposure since the 1980's, then their D3 levels have again became critically low and now what do we see?

Since the 1980's, in the northern latitudes, there has been an explosion of almost every disease or chronic condition known to man. Cancer, MS, autism, asthma, obesity, etc. Everything has skyrocketed since the 1980's! Much more on this later.

So, what is Vitamin D3? It is actually a steroid hormone that controls or affects at least 2,700+ genes by my count and likely many more. Many of these genes are involved in immune system regulation and tissue remodeling.

Originally it was found by the great Vitamin D3 researcher Dr Hollick, that Vitamin D3 directly affected 291 genes. He says:

"From his study -after giving Vitamin D3 to some volunteers and measuring their gene activity

there was at least a 1.5 fold inhibition of 82 genes (top ~30% of the heat map) whose expression was dramatically reduced and at least a 1.5 fold induction of 209 genes (bottom ~70% of the heat map) whose expression was significantly increased after supplementation with either 400 or 2000 IU of Vitamin D_3 for 2 months."

Recently there have been further studies describing how Vitamin D3 directly affects 700+ genes. Also, the higher the dosing of D3, the more genes that were affected.

However, it is now becoming known that not only does Vitamin D3 bind to VDR receptors at various gene sites, it also affects up to 2000 more genes by modifying the epigenetics of DNA (DNA methylation)-(these are things like methyl groups or proteins, that bind to DNA and alter the expression of genes by either inhibiting or increasing their rate of expression).

It is likely to be found that Vitamin D3 is involved in many more genetic pathways due to its major influence on signaling (non-coding) RNA molecules (such as lncRNA, siRNA, miRNA, piRNA, and snoRNAs for all you biochem fanatics) and their many gene controlling pathways. So, for now I am confident that 2,700+ genes being influenced by Vitamin D3 is a conservative estimate.

What is the big deal about this?

It turns out that Vitamin D3 is the master conductor of your immune and remodeling systems. At high levels it basically tunes up your immune system to be super vigilant and careful. And also prompts your remodeling system to conduct repairs and replacements of accumulated defective tissues.

The approximately 75% of all diseases (my estimate) that Vitamin D3 prevents and in most cases can cure are all caused by one problem- an out of tune immune/remodeling system! If your immune/remodeling system was operating perfectly, it would never attack good tissues by mistake and cause autoimmune diseases, and it would never accidentally ignore bad actors like bacteria, viruses, fungi and newly formed cancer cells. It would also repair all chronic defective tissues correctly and completely. In other words, you would be in perfect health and never get sick!

Now we have all been led to believe that the things that cause illness are out of our control, and in extreme cases this might be true. For example, if you drank a cup of radioactive isotopes, the insult would be so severe that likely no immune system could kill off all the cancer cells that would be generated from mutations and you would be overwhelmed. And then there are genetic diseases. Some are so severe that the immune/remodeling systems cannot overcome them as well. And then there are superbugs like the HIV virus that the human immune system has not yet evolved a way to kill it off. But these are the rare cases that do not apply to the great majority of people.

If you have autoimmune diseases that run in your family, you might believe that you are genetically destined to get an autoimmune disease. This I believe is false. As long as you keep your Vitamin D3 levels at the appropriate level for you, you will never get an autoimmune disease, even if there is a tendency for this in your family background (genes). I say this because amongst people with genetic tendencies to get a certain disease, not all of them do. So, what could be the difference amongst the predisposed between those who get the disease and those who don't? I believe it is not random chance but caused by differences in their immune systems that are controlled by Vitamin D3 levels.

Now your immune system, which destroys infectious bacteria, viruses, and fungi, also is intimately involved in your body's tissue remodeling system. In fact, you could say your immune system and your tissue remodeling system are two sides of the same coin.

Take macrophages for example, they are found throughout your body, and one of their main functions is to engulf and digest cellular debris, foreign substances, microbes, cancer cells, and anything else that does not have the type of proteins specific to healthy body cells on its surface in a process called phagocytosis. In addition to providing body wide immune functions, macrophages also have the following duties>>>

- muscle regeneration
- wound healing
- limb regeneration (in lower animals)
- iron homeostasis
- pigment retainment
- tissue homeostasis

Much of the same tool kit is used for both immune system and tissue remodeling functions.

Our bodies are constantly breaking down and rebuilding all our tissues all the time just at different rates-eyes, bones, skin, liver, blood, etc. When your immune system is out of whack, your remodeling system will likely be out of whack as well. This leads to wounds or injuries that do not heal properly like chronic wounds or things like plantar fasciitis, fistulas, cysts, chronic injuries etc. Over time if your remodeling system is not working well you can accumulate odd skin growths, odd pigmentation, various kinds of cysts, bone spurs, etc.

And even things like lesions on your nerve sheaths which occurs in MS, could be considered either an accidental attack by the immune system, or a failure of the tissue remodeling system to properly repair the lesions. Maybe it can be considered a double failure! So, to cure MS you have to stop the attack on the nerves by the immune system but also induce the remodeling system to properly repair the damage the immune system leaves behind. Luckily, high dose Vitamin D3 promotes both of these tasks quite well with no side effects! And you will soon see that 100,000's of people around the world have cured their MS with high dose D3 therapy of 1,000 IUs of D3 per kg. of body weight per day. High dose D3 also cures every other autoimmune disease it has been tried on so far. (Evidence to follow shortly).

Once your Immune/Remodeling System is in perfect working order by having the right amount of Vitamin D3 in your system orchestrating your immune/remodeling system genes like a symphony, you will-

-Never get an autoimmune disease such as MS, psoriasis, asthma, COPD, lupus, eczema, rheumatoid arthritis, acne, (see complete list at the end of this chapter).

-Never have tissue remodeling problems like bone spurs, chronic wounds, improperly healed injuries, as well as autism in newborns (more on this later).

-Almost NEVER catch any colds, or have any chronic infections like UTI's, bacterial, viral, or fungal infections.

-And the evidence strongly suggests you probably will never get cancer! (Overwhelming evidence to be presented shortly).

Note- my new definition of an autoimmune disease is basically any disease **not** caused by the bad actors such as infecting bacteria, fungi, viruses, parasites, or newly emerged cancer cells, that can be prevented OR cured with high dose Vitamin D3. Also, in general, autoimmune diseases are found at

45

a much higher rate in women than in men. So, to the list below we can add a few more like autism, acne, allergies, depression, diabetes-type II, COPD, etc.

I have compiled a list of all the autoimmune diseases as follows, and I will add a * next to the diseases I know for a fact have been cured by high dose Vitamin D3, others are just waiting for someone with the disease to do the self-experiment. It is interesting to note that the diseases with no asterisk tend to be less well-known diseases and rarer, and thus less likely to have been treated with a high dose Vitamin D3 experiment so far. All the more widespread autoimmune diseases have been cured or at least stopped from progressing with high dose Vitamin D3. Here is the list-any bold asterisked disease has been known to be cured by high dose Vitamin D3:

Rheumatoid arthritis   *
Psoriatic arthritis   *
Type 1 diabetes * (progression stopped with Vitamin D3 and fish oil).
Myasthenia gravis *
Celiac disease *
Hashimoto's thyroiditis *
Multiple sclerosis *
Psoriasis *
Systemic lupus erythematosus *

Lupus erythematosus *
Ulcerative colitis *
Crohn's disease *
Inflammatory bowel disease *
Scleroderma *
Granulomatosis with polyangiitis * See Wegener's below
Chronic fatigue syndrome *
Vitiligo *
Asthma *
Lichen planus * (topical D3)
Ankylosing spondylitis * (D3 with Borax as source of Boron)
Vasculitis *
Wegener's Disease * attack of vasculature of kidneys/lungs
Systemic scleroderma *
Dermatomyositis
Reactive arthritis
Sjögren syndrome
Graves' disease
Guillain–Barré syndrome
Primary biliary cholangitis
Antiphospholipid syndrome
Goodpasture syndrome
Neuromyelitis optica
Mixed connective tissue disease
Primary sclerosing cholangitis

Chronic inflammatory demyelinating
polyneuropathy
Lambert–Eaton myasthenic syndrome
Sarcoidosis
Raynaud syndrome
Kawasaki disease
Autoimmune polyendocrine syndrome
Autoimmune pancreatitis
Cold agglutinin disease
Balo concentric sclerosis
Optic neuritis
Gestational pemphigoid
Autoimmune inner ear disease
Palindromic rheumatism
Eosinophilic fasciitis
Susac's syndrome
Linear IgA bullous dermatosis
IgA nephropathy
IgG4-related disease
Behçet's disease
Sympathetic ophthalmia
Bullous pemphigoid
Autoimmune polyendocrine syndrome type 2
Relapsing polychondritis
Neutropenia
Undifferentiated connective tissue disease
Graves' ophthalmopathy
Cicatricial Pemphigoid
Eosinophilic granulomatosis with polyangiitis

Henoch–Schönlein purpura
Transverse myelitis
Cogan syndrome
Autoimmune oophoritis
Erythema nodosum
Autoimmune polyendocrine syndrome type 1
Pemphigus
Autoimmune hemolytic anemia
Morphea
Ord's thyroiditis
Aplastic anemia
Antisynthetase syndrome
Bickerstaff brainstem encephalitis
Hashimoto's encephalopathy
Thrombotic thrombocytopenic purpura
IPEX syndrome
Acute disseminated encephalomyelitis
Autoimmune Enteropathy
Opsoclonus myoclonus syndrome
Inflammatory demyelinating diseases of the central
nervous system
Drug-induced lupus erythematosus
CREST syndrome
PANDAS
Vogt–Koyanagi–Harada disease
Hughes–Stovin syndrome
Alopecia universalis

Plus+>

Diseases from my Expanded Definition of
Autoimmune Diseases-
Acne *
Allergies*
Birth complications-
Gestational Diabetes *
Pre-Eclampsia *
Infertility *
Low birth weight
SIDS
Premature Birth
COPD *
Costochondritis * (chest wall pain due to inflamed
cartilage)
Chronic Hives (urticaria) *
Diabetes Type 2 *
Depression *
Eczema *
Erectile Dysfunction *
Hypercholesterolemia *
Hypoglycemia *
Restless leg syndrome *
Congenital ichthyosis *
Parkinson's

Remodeling Diseases
AMD-Advanced Macular Degeneration *
Atherosclerosis (calcification of arteries) * (D3
with K2)

Autism * (Unusually large brain in infants never becomes normal)
Bone Spurs & hip clicks*
Bone & joint pain *
Blindness related to prior sinus infection *
Cataracts
Chronic Wounds *
Cracked heels-Excess Dead Skin on Feet *
Cysts *
Endometriosis *
Fistulas *
Glaucoma *
Heart Failure (heart enlargement) *
Hypertension *
Hypogonadism (low testosterone) *
Incontinence *
Nasal polyps *
Near/Far Sightedness *
Plantar fasciitis *
Scoliosis *
Skin tags *
Strokes *
Uterine Fibroids *
Varicose Veins *
Dementia – early onset

Hypo-Immune System Diseases – (failure to attack bad actors)
Yellow nail fungus (aka Onychomycosis) *
Common Cold *

Influenza *
Tuberculosis
Respiratory infections *
Urinary tract infections *
Bladder infections *
Sinus Infections *
Teeth infections *
Dental Cavities *
Intestinal infections *
Staph infections *
Ear infections*
All Cancers   > a qualified * (more on this in a
later chapter)

How is this possible? All of the above problems
seem like a separate disease or condition unrelated
to the others, but in fact they all track back to a
single cause, what I call an **unfocused
immune/remodeling system**. This is a broader
definition of autoimmune disease and basically
encompasses all diseases not specifically caused by
aging or new genetic mutations.

When your Vitamin D3 levels are too low for
optimal health, **<u>your immune system just
basically cannot see clearly</u>**, and it might attack
good tissues by accident, and allow bad actors like
viruses, bacteria, fungi, and newly formed cancer
cells to slide on by, mistaking them initially for
good tissues, or not being able to mount a rapid

enough defense to them to knock them out before they can do harm!

Humans are exposed to 600 to 1200 infectious bacteria and viruses every day, but getting sick from such contact tends to be rare. Most people catch a cold 2 to 4 times per year for viral colds. How is this possible? Your immune system usually spots and destroys infected cells before the virus can spread. When the 2700+ genes in your body that are controlled by Vitamin D3 get out of tune due to D3 deficiency, some virus infected cells can slip by and replicate fast enough before the immune system can respond. A Vitamin D3 revved-up immune system can apparently mount a very fast immune response, even to viral infections that a person has never been exposed to before. Why do I say this? Because from the 1,000+ high dose Vitamin D3 self-experiments I have heard about, there is one common theme that keeps popping up over and over. Those conducting high dose D3 experiments report over and over that they don't ever get colds anymore! Even when surrounded by contagious family members and co-workers.

I used to get about two bad colds a year until I started "high dose "Vitamin D3. Since then, I have only had one cold in the past 18 years since I started taking a minimum of 4000 IUs of Vitamin D3 for the first 10 of the last 18 years, and much higher doses for the last 8. And the time that I got the cold was when I had decided to take a break from D3 for a few months to clear out my system- that was a big mistake! You can search through my 1,000+ high dose Vitamin D3 case studies by using the search engine located at this link>

https://jefftbowles.com/vitamin-d3-cure-search-engine-can-d3-cure-your-disease-1000-case-studies/

Just type the disease or issue of interest in the search box and hit enter and get a long list of people's self-reports from all over the world that I have collected over the years. Why don't you start with the search term "cold"?

So apparently modern medicine has decided to protect our lazy immune systems from catching diseases like the flu; they expose us to a dead form of a virus before we encounter the live form. This allows our D3 deficient, slow motion immune systems to take their time to build up some immunity ahead of the time we are exposed to the virus.

However, if your immune system is revved up by Vitamin D3, you probably don't ever need any vaccinations. In fact, it has been shown that Vitamin D3 supplementation is 10X more effective at preventing the flu than the flu vaccine in Vitamin D3 deficient people! See my article on this at>>>

Lazy immune systems lead to frequently catching colds and the flu, but that is not the worst of it! Estimates vary widely, but one fact is agreed upon by almost all, that the human body produces cancer cells every day! Whether just 1 or in the 1,000's it is open for debate. But whatever the number, when your immune system is in tune and strengthened by high levels of Vitamin D3, the newly formed cancer cells simply get knocked off by the immune system before they can take hold and start replicating into a tumor. Only a lazy, out of focus immune system will make the mistake of ignoring a newly formed cancer cell. And ignoring a replicating cancer cell in the long run can be deadly because as the cancer replicates it picks up more and more mutations which in a way seem like they are programmed to turn the cancer cell into a new life form that becomes almost indestructible and then eventually sends out seeds to spread throughout your body (called metastasis).

In fact, my view of cancer is that it is actually a reversion to the original genetic program of the original single cell ancestors from which we evolved. Cancer cells can become immortal (this means they can keep dividing forever and never die of old age), and just continually reproduce (divide) and send out clones of themselves to colonize new areas.

Keep in mind that all the life forms you see around you, including humans, are all just a single cell that has evolved to replicate a great number of times into a large group of specialized versions of the original single cell that are all attached together. Every cell in your body is an identical copy of the single cell you began as, with just different controls placed on them to cause them to specialize. When those controls get out of whack in a cell it can become cancer.

Killing cancer cells when they first form is relatively easy for both doctors and your immune system-they really only become a problem after they pick up mutations to become immortal, harder and harder to kill, and spread throughout the body and eventually become out of reach of the immune system. If the immune system catches all newly formed cancer cells early, before they mutate down the path to immortality and metastasis, a spontaneously formed cancer cell will never be allowed to grow out of control. Basically, those whose immune systems are revved up by Vitamin D3 will NEVER get the disease of cancer in the course of a normal life. I will show evidence for this later-take my word for it now.

Basically, cancer is a disease of the immune system and nothing more. A highly focused D3-revved-up immune system should kill off all spontaneous cancer cells produced by the body, but what about those inborn genetic mutations that lead to cancer in some children like genetic retinoblastoma which causes 4% of all pediatric cancers)? The children with familial retinoblastoma aren't born with cancer but are diagnosed at the age of anywhere from 4 months to 4 years old, and usually both eyes are affected. But if their immune systems were vigilant enough, I expect that even familial retinoblastoma can be prevented with high dose Vitamin D3.

(Note- I was just thinking out loud when I wrote the prior sentence about D3 possibly being a preventive of retinoblastoma, I decided to research it and look what popped up)-

Ophthalmic Genet. 2002 Sep;23(3):137-56.
Vitamin D analogs, a new treatment for retinoblastoma: The first Ellsworth Lecture.
The main points of this study were:

- Researchers found Vitamin D receptors in retinoblastoma cells, suggesting potential for Vitamin D-based treatments.

- They tested Vitamin D and analogs in mouse models, finding effectiveness but also harmful hypercalcemia at therapeutic doses.

(I think they just need to add some Vitamin K2 to prevent these problems!)

- Two specific analogs, 16,23-D3 and 1α-OH-D2, showed effective tumor reduction with reduced toxicity.

- The mechanism involves increased p53-related gene expression and apoptosis.

- These promising results justify initiating clinical trials in children with retinoblastoma.

I later will devote a whole chapter on Vitamin D3 and cancer, and how the evidence is overwhelming that higher D3 levels dramatically reduce the chance of getting cancer to almost 0. And I also have a few cases to share with you about how high dose Vitamin D3 (50,000 IUs per day) have basically cured terminal cancer after the patients were sent home to die-much to the surprise of the doctors.

I have always believed that high dose Vitamin D3 should be able to cure cancer but the evidence has been sparse. I think this is mainly because most people are so scared of cancer when they are diagnosed that they don't try high dose D3 and just do whatever the doctor tells them. As for all the other diseases I have mountains of cases where high dose D3 has cured them -stay tuned. (If you are getting too skeptical to read further right now, take a break and cruise the

Search Engine For 1000+ Self-Reported Case Studies
of High-Dose Vitamin D3/K2 Experiments

(Pick a disease, any disease….)

Link>>> https://jefftbowles.com/vitamin-d3-cure-search-engine-can-d3-cure-your-disease-1000-case-studies/

Okay-what follows is what I consider overwhelming evidence that most human diseases are caused by Vitamin D3 deficiency. It is an abbreviated version of an article I wrote and published on my web site JeffTbowles.com. If you want to read the whole article in its entirety here is the link>>>>

https://jefftbowles.com/vitamin-d3-deficiency-causes-most-human-disease/

Overwhelming Proof That Vitamin D3 Deficiency Causes Most Human Diseases

August 2, 2019 <u>Jeff T Bowles</u>   (shortened version)

LATITUDE & THE INCIDENCE OF DISEASE:
OVERWHELMING PROOF THAT
VITAMIN D3 DEFICIENCY CAUSES
MOST HUMAN DISEASES
  It has been almost seven years since I published what was to become the best-selling book about Vitamin D3 in the world – translated into 10

languages so far. I thought I knew everything about Vitamin D3 back when the book was first published because in preparing for writing the book, I read or reviewed all 52,000 abstracts of science journal articles in the Pub Med science database that mentioned Vitamin D at that time.

However, in the last six years I have come up with a simple tactic to see if a disease is caused by Vitamin D3 deficiency and might be treatable with high-dose Vitamin D3-it has to do with the incidence of disease at various latitudes-more on this shortly. (I have heard from more than 1,000 people using high-dose Vitamin D3 to treat their various illnesses over the years, and have found that high-dose D3 is almost a miracle cure for up to 70 different diseases and conditions (and climbing) , including MS, lupus, depression, Crohn's disease, psoriasis, and many, many, more!) Of course, if you are new to Vitamin D3 your initial instinct would be to say:

"HA! If it sounds too good to be true – it probably is".

I assure you this is an exception to that rule as you will soon see and agree.

D3 is a hormone that tells your body that winter is over, and summer is here, and your body can stop hibernating and can go ahead and repair any incompletely repaired issues you have using all the resources. Most of us humans find ourselves in a state with chronically low Vitamin D3 levels all year long due to sun avoidance and use of sunscreen. I called this state – **the Human Hibernation Syndrome**. It is when your body acts as if it is preparing for a long winter famine, conserving resources required for complete repairs, slowing your metabolism, and urging you to conserve energy until the winter famine is over.

Vitamin D3 is referred to by some researchers as the bone and joint remodeling hormone and given that I have found how many people also notice its ability to repair the skin and soft tissues; I prefer to call it the all-tissue remodeling hormone.

One of my favorite examples of what Vitamin D3 can do comes in the form of a study they did on some rats. One group of rats received Vitamin D3 in their food while the other group did not. They then broke the poor rats' legs and then observed how they healed. The rats on a normal diet had healed legs where there was a large glob of extra bone around the break, like it was held together by a big ball of clay. The rats getting Vitamin D3 had perfectly healed fractures and you could not even notice where the break had been! This study says it all – what D3 can do for rat bones it can do for virtually any tissue in your body.

Basically, your body knows what shape it is supposed to be in. There is an exact blueprint of your entire body located in the DNA in the nucleus of each cell in your body. If your body has a chronic issue or incomplete repair, it is not an accident or loss of blueprint information. It just means your body is waiting until it gets the signal that conditions are right to do the repairs properly. That signal comes in the form of Vitamin D3. That condition is when summer returns and your Vitamin D3 levels go up and tell your body to go ahead and undo any partial repairs and to redo all the repairs perfectly using all resources necessary.

So that's it, now let's heap the overwhelming proof on you that is so easy to see. I will simply google-search a long list of diseases, along with the search term latitude, view the google images, and see if there are illustrations showing the incidence of a particular disease that varies in incidence with latitude. If the disease is found at lower rates near the equator and increases as you move away into latitudes with weaker sun, you can bet that it is a Vitamin D3 deficiency related disease!

Let's start with Multiple Sclerosis (my next case study article will be about the 1,000's of people all over the world who are curing their MS with high-dose Vitamin D3) Here is a graph I made from data from the data in a study: Multiple sclerosis vs latitude in 55 countries

Incidence of Multiple Sclerosis in 55 Countries-
X axis = Latitude
Y axis = Incidence of MS per 100,000 population

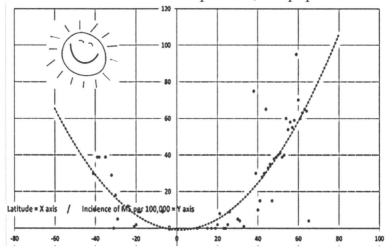

You will see this happy face distribution for virtually every autoimmune disease and every form of cancer as well as asthma. All you have to do is go to your favorite search engine, I like BING, and type in the disease of interest, then latitude then incidence and then look at the images that pop up. You will get almost the exact same "smiley face" graph that I showed you above.

The following is a list of various diseases that follow this exact same pattern. If you would like to see the original graphs that are on the internet, send me an email at or bannedcovidbook@gmail.com and I will send you a pdf file with lots of charts and images. Or you can just find them yourself on the internet-which is more fun.

Breast cancer
Colon Cancer
Leukemia
Multiple Myeloma: (white blood cell cancer)
All Other Cancers
Crohn's Disease and Ulcerative Colitis
Psoriasis
Lupus
Diabetes (Type 1-Juvenile)
Hypertension:
Tuberculosis:
Asthma-
Allergies and Eczema:
Depression & Suicide
Glaucoma
Alcoholism
Bi-polar Disease:
Schizophrenia-
Prevalence of schizophrenia within low (equator to 30 degrees), medium (30 to 60 degrees), and high (above 60 degrees) latitudes- While there was little variation found between these latitude ranges for females, **there was a significant increase of incidence and prevalence of schizophrenia for males the higher the latitude is**. There have been studies that show people with schizophrenia tend to be born during the winter/spring months. There are

also theories that say there could be a correlation between the amount of Vitamin D a pregnant woman has during the pregnancy of a fetus who then goes on to develop schizophrenia.

Autism-

A review of prevalence studies of Autism Spectrum Disorder by latitude and solar irradiance impact: A summary of 25 reports published between 2011 and 2016 using comparable diagnostic criteria **showed a tendency for the prevalence rates of ASD to be lowest in countries near the equator and for this rate to increase as the latitude increases.**

When viewing charts and graphs of diseases vs. latitude, some things to consider are:

- When you see an anomaly of a high prevalence area where low incidence should be expected, it often is caused by a larger proportion of dark-skinned individuals living in that area. Because it takes a lot more sun in darker skinned individuals to make Vitamin D3 than in lighter skinned ones.

- Keep in mind that sun avoidance is like a religion in the Middle East so you can see some unexpectedly high levels of disease at low latitudes.

In addition to the latitude effect, we have an
**INCREASING PREVALENCE SINCE 1980
EFFECT!**

What happened around 1980?
Many more of us started using sunscreen and/or
using more powerful sunscreens while also
avoiding the sun:

Introduction Date of Different Sunscreens and Melanoma Incidence by Year.

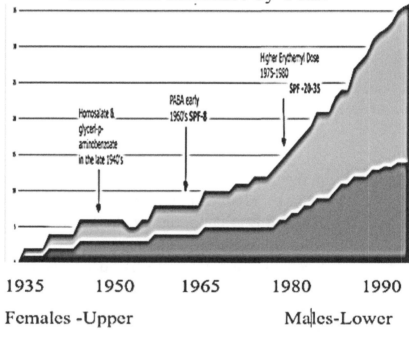

1935   1950   1965   1980   1990

Females -Upper   Males-Lower

It turns out that if you do not supplement with
Vitamin D3, you are more likely to DIE of skin

cancer (melanoma) if you use sunscreen than if you tan naturally. See my article:

Sunscreen Causes Skin Cancer, link>>>
https://jefftbowles.com/sunscreen-causes-cancer-vitamin-d-deficiency/

Studies have found that:
Sun avoidance is associated with earlier death: Over 15 years in a sun exposure study of the people who received **the most sun** exposure **96%** were alive after 15 years. The people with middle level exposure saw a **94%** survival rate and those with **the least sun** exposure saw only a **92%** survival rate after 15 years.

Darker skinned people need more and stronger sun to make the same amount of Vitamin D3 as lighter skinned people in the Northern latitudes – explaining the higher incidence of many diseases seen in darker skinned people living away from the equator.

Average Serum Vitamin D3 levels by Race
In America:
Blacks (Non-Hispanic)   **15.0 ng/mL**
Mexican Americans   19.7 ng/mL
Whites (Non-Hispanic)   25.9 ng/mL
In Africa:
African Blacks (Traditional Living) **46.1 ng/mL**

All of this sunscreen use and sun avoidance since at least the 1980's has led to an explosive rise in many diseases as you will see in the illustrations that follow:

Various Cancers

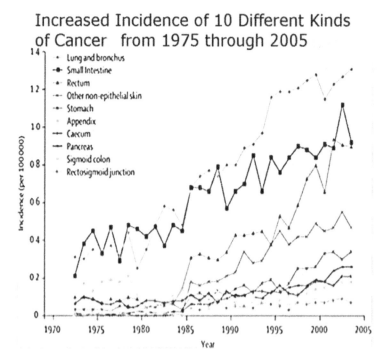

Increased Incidence of 10 Different Kinds of Cancer from 1975 through 2005

Autism

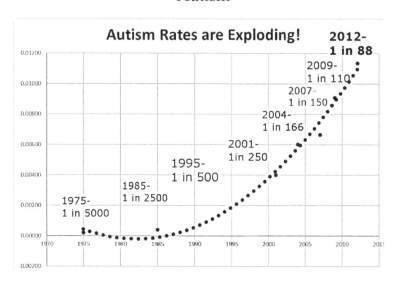

The Obesity Epidemic!

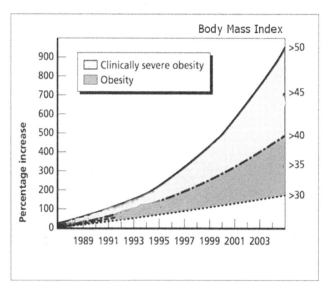

Type 1 (Juvenile) Diabetes:

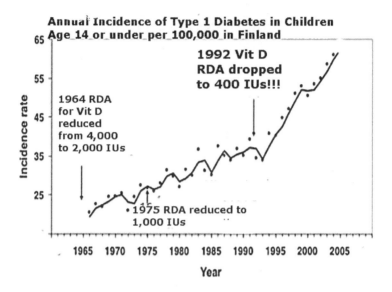

Annual Incidence of Type 1 Diabetes in Children Age 14 or under per 100,000 in Finland

1964 RDA for Vit D reduced from 4,000 to 2,000 IUs

1992 Vit D RDA dropped to 400 IUs!!!

1975 RDA reduced to 1,000 IUs

Incidence rate

Year

Childhood Cancer

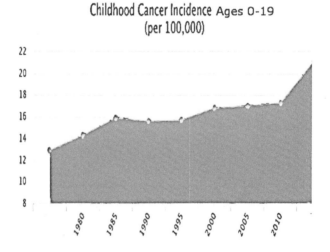

Childhood Cancer Incidence Ages 0-19
(per 100,000)

Thyroid Cancer – Exploding!

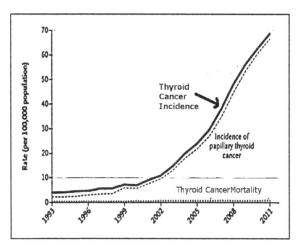

These charts go on and on; just do some searching for yourself on the internet- you can type in any disease and then the terms "incidence by year" and click on images and you will get graph after graph that looks just the same as the ones you have just seen. Some really dramatic ones include:

Malignant Melanoma
Food & Peanut Allergies
Celiac Disease (Gluten Intolerance)
Multiple Sclerosis is increasing
Parkinson's Incidence

So that's about it, the evidence, I believe is OVERWHELMING. And that is why I call Vitamin D3 deficiency the SMOKING CANNON for the cause of many diseases as well as the cause of the many epidemics of disease the world has been experiencing since the 1980's.

It turns out that there are quite a few gene variants that put you at risk for autoimmune diseases. They almost all are related to the Vitamin D3 receptor genes. The GREAT NEWS is that **most Vitamin D3 receptor defects can be overcome simply by taking much higher doses of Vitamin D3**.

PS- From time to time, as I find additional diseases or conditions that show a latitude effect and/or an increase after 1980 effect) I will add them here at the end of the article. These added diseases will likely be treatable with long-term, high-dose Vitamin D3 for 6 to 12 months (the time it takes to remodel one's tissues and immune systems back to normal).

Additional Diseases that follow the pattern of an increasing incidence vs latitude, and explosive rise since the 1980's.

For sake of brevity, I will just list the diseases added, email me at BannedCovidBook@gmail.com for a pdf with full text info and related charts and tables.

-Wegner's Disease and Vasculitis
-Migraines- There appears to be a latitude gradient suggesting it is Vitamin D3   related
-Vitiligo

-Ovarian Cancer
-Anaphylaxis- an acute allergic reaction to an antigen (e.g., a bee sting) to which the body has become hypersensitive
-Attention Deficit Hyperactivity Disorder
-Lung Cancer
-Prostate Cancer
-Dementia / Alzheimer's
-Parkinson's Disease
-Cholesterol Levels
-Cataracts
-Kawasaki Disease
-Chronic Wounds
-SIDS (Sudden Infant Death Syndrome)
-AMD (Advanced Macular Degeneration)
-ALS

OKAY So Now for Some Overwhelming Proof-

And keep in mind that later I will show you that various institutions from Harvard to Google to university research departments from all over the world do not want you to know these facts, and I believe are inadvertently and maybe even actively trying to suppress or discredit this information.

Now with most diseases what proof is there that these diseases are caused by Vitamin D3 deficiency? How about this, pick almost any disease on the list and I will show you cases where high dose Vitamin D3 **<u>cured</u>** the disease. (I say cured; others might call it being in complete remission. Some may say it is not a cure because those who are "cured" need to take D3 for the rest of their lives or the problem could come back.)

How can I show you where high dose D3 has cured somebody? I have been compiling cases for the high dose Vitamin D3 1,000+ case studies search engine for the last 8 years. And hearing from people from all over the world that have tried high dose D3 for everything from acne to ulcerative colitis to MS to psoriasis to COPD to blindness.

Let's start with the most convincing example first: Multiple Sclerosis.

I will now CONVINCINGLY show you that -

HIGH DOSE VITAMIN D3 CURES
MULTIPLE SCLEROSIS IN ABOUT 6 TO
10 MONTHS:

What follows is an abbreviated article I wrote for my website JeffTbowles.com about how the high dose Vitamin D3 has cured more than 100,000+ people around the world of their MS. If you want to read the full article here is the link>
https://jefftbowles.com/multiple-sclerosis-cure-by-high-dose-vitamin-d3/

The HIGH-DOSE Vitamin D3 CURE for Multiple Sclerosis –

Now SWEEPING THE PLANET

-Case Studies #14-
A Most Amazing Story of Dr. Coimbra and the 1,000's of his Patients around the world that have Been Cured of MS with High-Dose Vitamin D3 (Doses of 50,000, 100,000, 200,000 to as High as 1,000,000 IU of Vitamin D3 per day)

Have you heard the news? Big Pharma has just come out with a **miracle drug** for MS sufferers. The drug's name is ocrelizumab, and costs just **$65,000 per year**, and was shown to slow the decline in patients with primary progressive multiple sclerosis-the rarest form which no other drug has been able to affect, by 24%. The drug works by stamping out a class of immune cells, known as B cells, thought to play a major role in the disease. It also cuts time between relapses for those with relapsing MS by about 50%! Hmmm-no B cells? I wonder if there are any side effects?

Oh yeah>
upper respiratory tract infections,
infusion reactions (itching, rash, hives, redness, bronchospasm, swollen and sore throat, mouth pain, shortness of breath, flushing, hypotension, fever,

75

fatigue, headache, dizziness, nausea, and fast heart rate),
skin infections,
lower respiratory tract infections,
depression,
back pain, and
pain in the extremities
general swelling, Herpes outbreaks, and
cancer.
The National Multiple Sclerosis Society applauded the $65,000 price tag.

(I BET THEY DID!)

What if I told you there is a large and growing network of doctors around the world, associated with Dr. Coimbra, a pioneering Brazilian doctor who has been curing patients of MS and other autoimmune diseases with high-dose Vitamin D3 therapy for the past 7 years,

A SUPERIOR TREATMENT FOR MS AND BASICALLY A CURE – for a cost for the Vitamin D3, of as **little as $50 a year?**

What if I told you an ex-heavyweight professional boxer who once lost to the world champion Wladimir Klitschko and who contracted progressive primary MS (the worst kind) around the year 2000 and who was once wheelchair-bound, barely able to even move, and declining rapidly, is now learning to walk again after taking daily doses

76

of Vitamin D3 from 200,000 to as high as 1 million (recently) IU's for the last 7 years?

This is all true, and I am pretty sure most of you reading this have never heard a word about it from your doctor, and definitely not from Big Pharma! (I am sure they love the idea of millions of people shelling out $65,000 per year for their new drug for the rest of their lives!)

After we get through our first case of the MS-stricken boxer Zoran Vujicic, and the 1,000's of patients cured by Dr. Coimbra, I have testimonials from several other MS patients who swear to being cured via high dose Vitamin D3 therapy. I will add these cases to this article later.

Before we get into the interesting parts, let's just get an overview of what MS is all about:

MS affects an estimated 2.3 million people around the world, including about 400,000 people in the United States.

The four main types of MS are:

Clinically Isolated Syndrome (CIS)

Relapsing Remitting MS (RRMS)

Secondary Progressive MS (SPMS)

Primary Progressive MS (PPMS)

Relapsing remitting MS is the most common form of the disease. People with RRMS have acute attacks followed by periods of remission in which the disease doesn't progress. When this form becomes progressive, it's called secondary progressive MS.

The worst and rarest kind of MS is called primary progressive (PPMS) which makes up about 10-15% of MS sufferers. Once it starts, it does not get better, there are no remission periods. It is just straight downhill, or coasting, until complete paralysis and death. Zoran Vujicic has this kind.

What differentiates PPMS from the relapsing forms is that while active progression may stop temporarily, the symptoms do not resolve. In relapsing forms, the symptoms may actually improve or return near to where they were before the most recent relapse. Another difference is that there's not as much inflammation in PPMS compared to relapsing forms. Because of this, many of the drugs that work for relapsing forms do not work for PPMS or SPMS. Also, with PPMS, there are fewer lesions in the brain and more in the spinal cord. The progression of symptoms can worsen over a few months or several years.

What is an MS lesion? It is kind of like a pimple or ulcer on the sheath of tissue that covers one's nerves or brain cells. It is like an electrical wire loses some of its insulation and starts to short circuit.

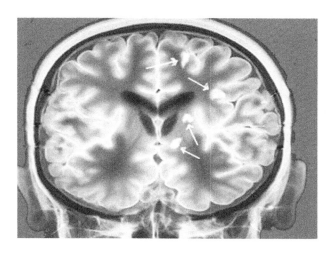

An MRI of MS lesions

MS is more common in Caucasians than in other ethnic groups. Although relapsing forms of MS (as almost all autoimmune diseases) are more common in women than in men, both sexes get PPMS at about the same rate. PPMS tends to occur about 10 years later in life than the relapsing forms of MS.

With 160 cases of MS per 100,000 inhabitants, Norway ranks seventh in MS disease prevalence worldwide, behind only Canada, Denmark, Sweden, Hungary, Cyprus and the United Kingdom, (according to the Multiple Sclerosis International Federation). (Notice the high latitudes where the sun is weak and Vitamin D3 levels are low for most of these countries-this will be important later).

(this illustration omitted in paperback-please see eBook or request pdf at BannedCovidBook@gmail.com)

Notice how MS is more prevalent where the sun is weakest (and thus Vitamin D3 levels are lower-Vitamin D3 is made when strong sun hits your skin).

Oddly, even though MS sounds like a terrible, life-threatening disease, most sufferers of MS can live quite a long time and have an average age of death of only 7 years or so younger than normal people!

However, the symptoms can be bad to horrible, including complete paralysis amongst those with PPMS. Milder symptoms include dizziness, vision and cognitive problems, fatigue, bowel and bladder problems, sexual issues, motor problems, and pain.

Well now for the GOOD NEWS!>>

Dr. Coimbra and his 5,000+ patients – Dr. Cicero Galli Coimbra is a Brazilian Neurologist, Professor and Researcher who has become popular for treating Multiple Sclerosis and autoimmune disease with high doses of Vitamin D3 combined with a combination of other supplements and diet recommendations. Dr. Coimbra does not claim to

cure MS [some of his patients will tell
you differently] but he has proven that his treatment
does stop its progression.

Here is a great link to testimonials of many of Dr.
Coimbra's patients>>

http://www.thisisms.com/forum/coimbra-high-
dose-vitamin-d-protocol-f57/topic27155-105.html

You will find many testimonials similar to this one
by Kory:

(this illustration omitted in paperback-please see
eBooks or request pdf from
BannedCovidBook@gmail.com)

Re: Multiple Sclerosis Testimonials (Coimbra
Protocol)

Kory's Testimonial
This is Kory Carreño, from **Peru**. Many of us,
patients of Dr. Coimbra, have followed Kory's
story with the Coimbra Protocol and her struggle to
go to Brazil in 2012 and start the treatment with
high doses of Vitamin D. This is what Kory has
recently shared with our FB groups:

Hello, my name is Kory Carreño, I am from Lima /
Peru, and had my first MS symptoms in 1999. I
went from one doctor to another, always ending up
in psychiatrists, until I had half of my body
paralyzed in 2004 and, after an MRI, the doctors

said I possibly had MS. They did not prescribe any treatment, and after several weeks I ended up losing function of the other half of my body. I was a quadriplegic, I was admitted to the hospital and received 1000 mg per day of methyl prednisone for 15 days – dose sufficient to lead to death. I was just devastated. At that time, I was living in Bolivia and they sent me back to Peru because in Bolivia they knew nothing about the disease.

In Peru, they treated me with AVONEX for three years. Besides the side effects, I had 3 to 4 had relapses per year, and it used to take me 2 to 3 months to recover, and hence came another relapse. I was very tired, but I kept going for my son. This medication only hurt me, my body created a resistance to the interferon, and its use has caused me leukopenia (reduction in the number of leukocytes in the blood) and my hemoglobin dropped to 6.7, that is, I became anemic. The doctors discontinued the treatment and I had more relapses, one after the other without interruption. I began to despair because I started to be dependent on a wheelchair, I needed a probe to feed me and a cervical collar to keep my neck up. Doctors disillusioned me, but I refused to accept that I had to stay that way.

With the help of friends, I traveled to the US in search of a clinical trial, but they said that I had to use Copaxone. To buy this medication we had to do many fundraising, etc. With Copaxone I had a relapse a year for two years, I got a little stronger and started searching the internet. But the drugs I used all those years caused me cervical cancer. I got my uterus removed and thank God the cancer was eliminated, but I had another big relapse.

In 2012 I met a patient with MS who told me about the Vitamin D Protocol (thank God, who is always behind everything bringing Angels to our lives, because He loves us more than anything in the world!) And through this person I met Yara Correa, a patient from Brazil, and she introduced me to this INCREDIBLE Protocol. I watched Dr. Cicero's videos and realized that that was what I was looking for. I could not believe it was exactly what I had asked the Lord Jesus: that I could stop mistreating my body with chemicals and not experience side effects anymore, no longer inject cortisone, no longer have relapses and leave my son at home without knowing if or how I'd return. I was blessed to have friends and family who moved heaven and earth for me to travel to Sao Paulo, and Yara offered me all the support I needed in Brazil.

With 8 months of treatment, I was very happy and stopped the injections (Copaxone). No relapses and many improvements. Unfortunately, the doctors found two tumors in my ovaries, which due to negligence they had not removed in the previous surgery. When I was hospitalized, Dr. Cicero (through Yara) was always attentive. I continued taking my dose of 60,000 IU per day and my multivitamins. Everything went well, the 2 tumors were benign, and the most FABULOUS thing of all was that I had no relapses. After 9 months of treatment, I got married!

After 4 years of treatment, I'm now enjoying life with my family, and many of my disabilities have disappeared. I can go horse riding, I can walk alone, without support, lead a normal life without pain, and I do not wake up tired in the morning. Blessed Vitamin D and Dr. Cicero.

I had a friend who died as a result of various experimental treatments for patients with MS, and they are so harmful that they can lead to death. That's why now I want everyone to know about this protocol. I wish my friend had a little bit of the luck I had, but God knows all things. I tried everything that was "natural" before this Protocol: bees' stings, raw diet, other diets, but I can tell you that Dr. Cicero Coimbra and the Vitamin D Protocol were placed by God to save lives and we have to announce it to the world.

Here is a before and after picture of another D3 success story – John Ottwell, (with PPMS) before, and at day 165 on the protocol. (his recovery was amazingly fast as compared to Zoran's)

(this illustration omitted in paperback-please see eBook or request pdf at BannedCovidBook@gmail.com)

(this illustration omitted in paperback-please see eBook or pdf)

Dr. Coimbra has treated himself or through his network of affiliated doctors more than 5,000 MS patients with a success rate he claims of 95%. There are possibly hundreds of testimonials all over the internet that are easy to find so I will not add any more of Coimbra's patients. You can even see him/them in many YouTube videos like this one>>

Vitamina D – Por uma outra terapia (subtitled)

https://youtu.be/erAgu1XcY-U

Or How about the first US patient to use the Coimbra protocol under a US doctor's care-Jennifer Butler's story>

Jennifer Butler about her journey with MS and the Coimbra Protocol

https://youtu.be/s5WyGNhdt8M

If you have any doubts about how far and wide high-dose Vitamin D3 therapy for MS is spreading just take a look at the many Facebook groups in many different languages devoted to the topic>>

Coimbra protokol, visoke doze vitamina D3 – MS i druge autoimune bolesti – 9,000 members

PROTOCOLO COIMBRA – Vitamina D para Esclerose Múltipla e Doenças Autoimunes 28,000 members

Vitamina D3 – Dose Fisiológica 706 members

Protocolo Coimbra – Esclerose Multipla e Outras Doenças Auto Imunes 10,000 members

Espondilite Anquilosante & D3 Vitamina 2,000 members

Vitamin D3 – Čudežni hormon! Zaustavimo multiplo sklerozo! 1,000 members

CoimbraProtokollen Norge – D-vitamin for MS og autoimmune tilstander 800 members

Protocolo Coimbra México - Vitamina D3 Para Enfermedades Autoinmunes 345 members

O tratamento com vitamina D do Dr. Cícero Coimbra – Portugal 15,000 members

Vitamina D – Emodieta- protocollo Coimbra…Guarire dalle autoimmunità 7,000 members

Visoki dozi na Vitamin D za avtoimuni bolesti – Coimbra protokol 700 members

Multiple Sclerosis – Vitamin D 1,000 members

Vitamina D – Brasil 37,000 members

Coimbra Vitamin D Protocol for MS & Autoimmune Disorders 6,000 members

One of the most interesting Dr. Coimbra related sites on the web has before and after pictures of his MS patients MRIs like this one.

(this illustration omitted in paperback-please see eBook or request pdf)

Now I would like to tell you about one special case of the one MS patient, Zoran Vujicic, who contacted me from the country of Montenegro a number of years ago, after reading my book on high-dose Vitamin D3 therapy.

Up until the year 1999, Zoran was a heavyweight professional boxer. In that year he fought against Wladimir Klitschko who would eventually become the heavyweight champion of the world. Unfortunately, Zoran lost, but that was just the beginning of a bad turn in his life.

Soon after he developed PPMS and eventually became wheelchair bound for many years. Sometime around 2015, Zoran read my book which was difficult for him because his first language is Serbian. However, after making it through the book he decided to give high-dose Vitamin D3 therapy a try. And what a try he did. He was quickly taking a dose as high as 200,000 IU per day. But he was doing it in an intelligent way, by carefully monitoring his blood calcium levels on a monthly basis to make sure they stayed in the normal range. Zoran also was taking high-dose Vitamin K2 which was promoted in my book because it makes taking Vitamin D3 safer by catalyzing the incorporation of blood calcium into one's bones.

You see the only real danger of taking too high a dose of Vitamin D3 is that it could cause the release of too much calcium into your blood which could lead to kidney stones, improper calcification of soft tissues, nausea, rapid weight loss, and other bad things. But keep in mind this hypercalcemia effect of Vitamin D3 is **much rarer** than most doctors would lead you to believe. The good news is, that unlike many Big Pharma drugs, **these potential adverse consequences of high-dose Vitamin D3 are easy to reverse** by simply stopping intake of D3 to allow your D3 levels to come down. And unlike with Big Pharma's drugs, cancers, infections, and death are not potential side effects associated with Vitamin D3.

Zoran's treatment regimen differed from the Coimbra protocol in that he also took large doses of Vitamin K2 with his high-dose Vitamin D3. The Vitamin K2 recharges the proteins that take calcium out of your blood and put it back into your bones. Dr. Coimbra agrees that K2 works at removing calcium from the blood at lower levels of D3 but disputes the idea that at very high doses of D3 that

K2 can have any effect. Zoran may be proving this idea incorrect.

Zoran maintained the 200,000 IU per day for a couple of years and found that it completely halted the progression of his MS. However, after those few years, he was no longer satisfied with this result and embarked on his own experiment of higher and higher doses of D3. At the time of this writing, he claims to be taking 500,000 to 1 million IU's of D3 per day with lots of K2 and magnesium. **Amazingly his blood tests keep coming back with his calcium in the low range of the scale!** If anyone is to try what seems like a very dangerous treatment dosage, you should definitely go up gradually, and get your blood calcium checked VERY OFTEN…maybe every 2 weeks for a while. And if you feel nauseous and start losing weight that would be a sign that hypercalcemia was being triggered and you would have to stop and adjust your dosage.

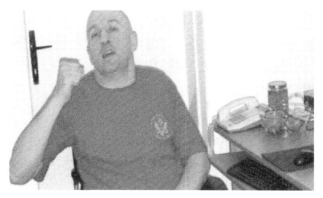

<u>Zoran walks again with friends; help-2019.</u>

Here is a link to a video of him standing by himself>>
https://www.facebook.com/messages/t/zoran.vujicic.5

Zoran's case differs from those who follow Coimbra's protocol in that he is taking high-dose Vitamin K2 and does not follow any rules about restricting calcium intake.

Coimbra suggests that his patients should take only about 1,000 IU of D3 per kg of body weight per day, and he feels Vitamin K2 has no effect at such high levels of D3. He also instructs his patients to strictly avoid calcium-rich foods and drink an extra liter or 2 per day of water to wash the calcium out of one's blood. **<u>Zoran does not drink extra water, nor does he avoid calcium, but he does take large doses of Vitamin K2 with his D3-lkely a more fun lifestyle than not being to ever eat pizza again!</u>**

In addition to the many testimonials you can read about Dr. Coimbra's patients on the internet, you can also use the Vitamin D3 1,000+ case studies search engine

Link> https://jefftbowles.com/vitamin-d3-cure-search-engine-can-d3-cure-your-disease-1000-case-studies/

Search Engine-Can D3 Cure your Disease? 1000+ Case Studies

and find even a few more testimonials from people treating themselves like these>>

Hi Jeff,

Hope you are having a good summer Just to jog your memory, last year I wrote to you after reading your books. My 35-years old husband, J*** was newly diagnosed with **MS**. You told me about Dr. Coimbra's protocol for **MS** at the time.

After the tip from you, J*** said goodbye to conventional medical immediately and started the high-dose Vitamin D protocol with a doctor trained in it. He's been on the protocol for 8 months now and we are very happy with the results. His blood reports show no inflammation and the last MRI scan showed no new or active lesions. He still has the old lesions that will probably take a few years to go away, but that can take its own sweet time. We do not mind because it takes time to heal and he is healing very nicely so far. Although he sometimes has some numbness and tingling, he has had no relapses. He is full of energy; you know well how the high doses of Vitamin D give you good energy levels and better quality of day to day life. J*** manages a job where he works offshore in long shifts (12 hours or more) when he is onboard the subsea rig where he works. Simultaneously he is also in the middle of his engineering studies and of course, the household calls his attention too as we have 2 little girls. We are otherwise two physically active people who like skiing, sailing, hiking, camping in nature etc. He is able to do all of this like he did before. Crazy to think that he lives such an active life that normal people don't have the energy for while having **MS** only by taking high doses of Vitamin D and a few other vitamins. This is miraculous!

I only wanted to update you and keep you in the loop. Jaro will be going for an MRI in Oct-Nov period so we will see if there is any change in the liaison, I will let you know.

Keep doing the good work of spreading the news on Vitamin D, I owe you and so many others for introducing us to the miraculous of "dangerously high-dose" Vitamin D. Take care and enjoy the summer.

Best wishes
M*****

5.0 out of 5 stars must read for those suffering with **MS**

By J. Crawford on February 28, 2014

Read this in 2 days, I was fascinated. I've had **MS** way longer I know than 20 years (diagnosed 17 ago). I've started high dose D3 therapy 2 weeks ago. I'm not saying I'm CURED, but I can notice a difference in my balance and pain level already and I'm hopeful for further improvement. Read this with an open mind. I'm really happy with, and excited that I found this book!

Here is the follow-up email from Manisha re **MS.** She suggests if you start D3 immediately upon diagnosis you can nip it in the bud, and one should skip conventional treatment altogether!!

Ok I have truncated this article for brevity you can read the rest of it at my website link, it has more testimonials from the search engine and a large update on Zoran >>>>> https://jefftbowles.com/multiple-sclerosis-cure-by-high-dose-vitamin-d3/

Oh, wait here is another interesting blurb from the article>

(this illustration omitted in paperback-please see eBook or request pdf)

Between 1989 and 2006, the incidence of MS in Iran increased more than 8X

One striking example of the rise in MS is in Iran where, after the Islamic revolution in 1979, women were compelled by law to wear the veil outdoors together with clothing covering most of the body. Between 1989 and 2006, the incidence of MS in Iran increased more than eight-fold, from an incidence of about one case in 100,000 to nearly one in 10,000 in the city of Isfahan.

"The Islamic revolution can potentially explain the observed increase in MS incidence in Iran in just over 30 years," said Dr, Ramagopalan. "Veiled women have lower Vitamin D levels compared to unveiled women, giving an increased risk of low Vitamin D in pregnancy which can account for the increase in MS."

Okay so back to the overwhelming evidence.

The article is pretty convincing right? High dose Vitamin D3 can and does cure MS. And long with the chart that shows MS increases the further you move away from the equator the rates of MS go up strongly suggests that higher doses of Vitamin D3 can prevent MS. All studies show this is true, so you don't really have to rely on the chart. However, once you see the same pattern popping up for almost all other diseases, you can pretty much connect the dots and eventually realize that almost all diseases are caused by Vitamin D3 deficiency and can be cured by high dose Vitamin D3.

Does the MS model apply to most other diseases? Why yes it does. Go back and review the Overwhelming proof article you just read, and you will find most every disease you can think of showing the same latitude/incidence chart pattern as MS.

Now as far as high dose Vitamin D3 curing every autoimmune disease known to man, I have lots of articles on most of the diseases that always include several detailed self-reports of how D3 cured their diseases.

Rather than print them all here you can go to my website: JeffTbowles.com and look through the blog posts. You will find many dozens of articles about specific diseases. Below is a list of the articles available on the blog post sorted by number of views so far-. You see the titles are self-explanatory in most cases, high dose D3 cures this or that disease. There are many of them to read and they all indicate the same thing-**high dose Vitamin D3 cures all autoimmune and lazy immune system conditions.**

LINKS TO- All Articles Available In these Blog Pages

Ranked by Popularity

(If theses links are active in the eBook you can just put your cursor on an article title and hit enter and it should take you there)

Otherwise go to this link for this active links list>

https://jefftbowles.com/articles-available-in-these-blog-pages-ranked-by-popularity/

March 12, 2019 Jeff T Bowles

(this illustration omitted in paperback-please see eBook or request)

Title	Views
Vitamin D3 Case Study #3: Plantar Fasciitis of 3 years – Completely cured in 2 weeks!	13,295
OVERWHELMING PROOF THAT VITAMIN D3 DEFICIENCY CAUSES MOST HUMAN DISEASES	7,945
The HIGH-DOSE Vitamin D3 CURE for Multiple Sclerosis – Now Sweeping the Planet – Case Studies #14	5,550
Search Engine-Can D3 Cure your Disease? 1000+ Case Studies	5,425
Longer Term High-Dose Vitamin D3 Therapy Cures Asthma-Case Studies #10	4,311
The 6 Changes in Lifetime Hormone Levels that Cause Aging – And How to Easily Reverse Them!	4,134
Case Study #9 – A Doctor Cures His	3,987

and has cured blindness in one eye caused by thrombosis,

Now the major disease category that you will not yet see in a big way on the list is the most feared disease of all- cancer. I believe I know the reason for this and will address it in a later chapter. What I can say now is that I do have several cases to share with you where high dose Vitamin D3 (50,000 IUs per day) did cure or at least put into remission a number of cancers. So, if we don't have a large number of cancer cures via D3 to show you, how can we make the statement that taking higher doses of Vitamin D3 should prevent you from ever getting cancer.

There is lots of evidence that shows the cancer is prevented by high dose D3 which you saw in chart after chart, graph after graph in the "overwhelming proof" article Cancer apparently rarely occurs at the equator where the sun is the strongest, and increases in incidence the further you move away from the hot sun. You also saw how almost all kinds of cancer are increasing in incidence since the 1980's when sun avoidance and sunscreen became the rule for "good health" HA! If you want to review the article again, here is the link>

https://jefftbowles.com/vitamin-d3-deficiency-causes-most-human-disease/

What Doctors and Vitamin D Researchers

Do not Know or Pretend to Not Know About Vitamin D3

I recently undertook a task to see exactly what was going on in the field of Vitamin D research. I was wondering how could millions of doctors, and huge numbers of Vitamin D researchers, and everyone in Big Pharma and at the FDA be so wrong about Vitamin D3?!

How are they wrong?

-They mostly **all believe low doses of Vitamin D3 are actually high, dangerous doses!** For example, many doctors believe that 2,000 to 10,000 IU's of Vitamin D3 are high doses bordering on dangerous, when an average adult sunbathing in the summer sun in Finland, a very northerly location with weak sun, for just ½ hour can make 20,000 IUs of D3 in their skin! 2,000 IUs of D3 is actually too low a dose to do anything-yet many researchers use this dose in massive studies calling it "high dose". Take Harvard's massive years long VITAL study of D3 with 20,000+ participants for example. They look at disease after disease and say "high dose D3" has no effect! Is this innocent ignorance or intentional misinformation? It sure would be in Big Pharma's and modern medicine's interests to relegate high dose Vitamin D3 to the dust bin so they can

103

continue on selling their outrageously priced drugs and medical services. HMMMM!

-Some doctors and researchers think that Vitamin D2 and D3 are interchangeable and of equal efficacy. Vitamin D2 is an inferior plant-synthesized version of the hormone Vitamin D3 with important chemical differences that make D2 less effective than D3 and having negative side effects, hypercalcemia in particular! **There are still researchers and doctors using Vitamin D2 when the practice should be outlawed!**

In a 2017 study titled How much is too much? Two contrasting cases of excessive Vitamin D supplementation, the authors present two contrasting cases of high-dose Vitamin D intake, showcasing the potential impact of Vitamin D source. Both patients took substantial daily doses for over a year, 50,000 for D2 and 40,000 for D3, but with drastically different outcomes. The 75-year-old man, taking Vitamin D2 (ergocalciferol), suffered severe toxic effects like hypercalcemia with blood levels of 243 ng/ml, while the 60-year-old woman taking Vitamin D3 (cholecalciferol) remained asymptomatic despite even having higher serum Vitamin D levels (479 ng/ml). This suggests a potential difference in individual response based on the type of Vitamin D taken.

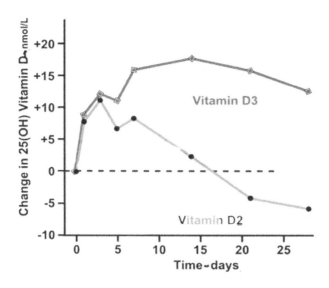

-Most doctors and researchers think Vitamin D3 is actually toxic! When in **fact it is completely nontoxic**-D3 is merely information supplied to your DNA to tune up your immune system and remodel your tissues. The only potential harm from D3 comes from excess calcium in your blood or exacerbation of an existing magnesium deficiency. Vitamin D3 itself is completely nontoxic! And excess calcium in the blood can be easily prevented by supplementing with Vitamin K2 and occasional blood monitoring of calcium. Magnesium deficiency can be corrected with careful magnesium supplementation.

-Doctors and researchers have extremely **exaggerated fears about the possibility that "high dose" Vitamin D3 can cause hypercalcemia** and is dangerous, when this is extremely rare and almost never happens. Most cases of hypercalcemia (which are very rare) were likely to occur with High Dose Vitamin D2 as opposed to using Vitamin D3.

-Doctors and researchers do not know that higher doses of Vitamin D3 will rapidly use up your magnesium stores and that magnesium supplementation with high dose D3 is a must. Then they see various symptoms of magnesium deficiency like increased risks of falls, confusion, lethargy, arrhythmias, panic attacks, etc. and blame it on the D3 when it is actually an underlying subclinical magnesium deficiency (hypomagnesia) being exacerbated and unveiled in the patient.

-Doctors and researchers generally do not know that any cases of hypercalcemia associated with "high dose" Vitamin D3 use is caused not by the Vitamin D3 itself, but by the fact that **higher levels of Vitamin D3 cause your body to use up Vitamin K2 stores** that are necessary to take calcium out of your blood and soft tissues and put it back in your bones.

-Most doctors and researchers **have no idea of the proper dosing level and schedule of Vitamin D3.**

Because Vitamin D3 is stored in the fat cells for long periods, dosing protocols are all over the place. Some medical practitioners think it is fine to give their patients a large dose of Vitamin D3 just once a month! From 100,000 to 300,000 IUs and more. And they are perplexed when they see an increase in the number of falls in their patients receiving bolus injections as opposed to regular daily dosing. Why?

Because they have no idea that high dose Vitamin D3 will exacerbate an underlying magnesium deficiency, and three symptoms of magnesium deficiency are dizziness, falls, and fainting! On the other hand, most practitioners who prescribe daily Vitamin D3 dosing prescribe amounts that are so low that they are **guaranteed to be ineffective.** Consider that an adult can make 20,000 IU's of D3 from ½ hour of whole-body summer sunbathing in Finland! And they think 1,000 or 2,000 IUs a day is going to make much difference. Preposterous!

With these problems in mind I have come up with a list of new guidelines for Vitamin D3 dosing for doctors and Vitamin D3 researchers-

> -**Never give a patient Vitamin D2.** It is far inferior to Vitamin D3 for the intended purpose. Vitamin D2 is the hormone that plants make and use, it is chemically different than the hormone animals make in

their skin or on their fur when exposed to sunlight which is Vitamin D3. Vitamin D3 is much more effective, has a much stronger effect than D2 and a much longer half-life. Just stop using Vitamin D2 for anything! It is hereby banned!

-Eliminate the practice of bolus injections of high doses of Vitamin D3. **Prescribe only daily doses of Vitamin D3** for patients and test subjects, doing anything else makes all data comparisons completely worthless. If we can all agree to daily dosing of Vitamin D3 we can then have a much more workable data set to work with by limiting the treatment to a single variable- the dose. Also, by eliminating the periodic bolus injection protocol we will also drastically **reduce the risk of falls** caused by high dose Vitamin D3 aggravating an underlying magnesium deficiency.

-Never prescribe Vitamin D3 without **also giving the patient magnesium and Vitamin K2.** To do so would be malpractice as we will see in later chapters.

-**NEVER give extra calcium** to a patient receiving higher doses of Vitamin D3. The main possible danger of Vitamin D3 which practitioners are so wary of is hypercalcemia-so why on earth would you give a patient extra calcium with Vitamin D3? You should only do this if you also have them supplementing with significant amounts of Vitamin K2 to put the excess calcium in the blood back into the bones. Osteoporosis is likely better treated with Vitamin K2, magnesium and boron dosing as opposed to calcium. Most diets contain plenty of calcium, so throwing more calcium at the bones is not going to fix the osteoporosis and more likely to cause soft tissue calcification problems.

-One dose fits all is not a logical or smart way to gauge the effects of Vitamin D3. I have found that two people of the same weight can take a certain dose of Vitamin D3 and have two completely different changes in the blood level of their D3. For example, I know of two people, about the same weight, they both started taking 20,000 IU of D3 per day. One's blood level of D3 skyrocketed to 180+ ng/ml while the other's blood level barely budged from 30 to 50 ng/ml. We call them high responders and low responders. The reasons for this are not yet clear, but it might have to do with the differing levels of magnesium in their systems. Anyway, the highly preferred way **to conduct research or monitor patients is to follow their blood levels for D3 and shoot for a particular blood level and adjust the dose of D3 to achieve it on a case-by-case basis.** Yes, it is more work, but it is the only way to use D3 properly.

-Based on my review of "high dose "Vitamin D3 experiments to be discussed in the next chapter, I would like to propose that **no studies of Vitamin D3 be conducted with any dose less than 10,000 IUs of D3 per day on average per adult patient.** This is barely the amount of D3 one can make in their skin by summer sunbathing for 15 minutes! Also, a recent review of how the daily recommended daily allowance was calculated by the esteemed Institute of Medicine (IOM) found a statistical error **that led to an underestimation of the proper daily dose by 90%! A decimal point error!!!** Here is the abstract from that study, you can read the full study as Appendix A at the end of this book or at this link>>>> https://www.ncbi.nlm.nih.gov/pmc/articles/PMC5541280/

OOPS! Just an innocent little decimal point error and the United States has accidentally spent about 80% to 90% more on health care than was necessary for decades! Was it really just an innocent error? How did it stay unnoticed for so long? These are obvious questions everyone must ask!

Dimitrios T. Papadimitriou wrote a review article titled The Big Vitamin D Mistake; his conclusions can be summarized as follows:

Finland's vitamin D milk boost is tied to a dramatic type 1 diabetes drop! But don't blame sunshine alone - research points to a major blunder in recommended intake! The original RDA was off by a whopping factor of 10, meaning most people need way more than the measly 600 IU promoted by the Institute of Medicine. Studies show optimal levels may require daily doses around 8,000 IU for young adults and beyond! Public health needs to rethink these outdated recommendations to protect against widespread vitamin D deficiency and potentially other health woes.

From my experience of reviewing over 1,000+ high dose Vitamin D3 self-experiments it has become clear that **to cure chronic diseases one needs to achieve a blood level of Vitamin D3 of 125-150 ng/ml or higher (=375 nmol/L).** The appropriate dose is unique to each individual patient, the practitioner needs to find the dose that achieves target blood level. This dose may greatly vary between individuals.

Anything less than 150 ng/ml will likely not work. And this is not just my observation, but also was observed by Dr. Harald Schelle of Germany who is an ophthalmologist who wrote his own book on how he switched to using high dose Vitamin D3 in his practice to treat all his patients. (Book Title- Vitamin D3 High dosage The Alternative to the previous therapy of Glaucoma: Newest Findings revolutionize Cancer prophylaxis+ General Therapy Ophthalmology Wearing of Contact lenses).

The current reference range in the US for "normal" levels of blood-Vitamin D3 is 30 – 100 ng/ml. But where does this range come from? It is just the results of sampling the blood from a population of, for the most part, Vitamin D3 deficient people that live up north far away from the equator. It is the range of D3 levels of a Vitamin D3 deficient population. Doctors assume that the average person in this group has plenty of Vitamin D3 – but I say this is incorrect. For example, a summer lifeguard in Florida often has blood levels of 125 ng/ml. But he or she achieves these blood levels by sitting in relatively weak sun (compared to the equatorial sun) usually under an umbrella wearing a hat and sporting zinc oxide on the nose. If you went to the doctor and he or she saw your blood level of D3 was 125 ng/ml the doctor might have a fit and tell you to stop all D3 intake and look for signs of toxicity! This is ridiculous!

The one major thing that is **missing** from the Vitamin D3 dosing debate is a good set of **comprehensive sunbathing studies**! If we knew how much Vitamin D3 is made in the skin by sunbathing 1 hour, 2 hours, 3 hours, 4, etc. we would quickly learn what evolution deems a normal dose of Vitamin D3. And I can guarantee you that it is way more than 2,000 IU per day as used in most large-scale Vitamin D3 studies. After years of looking at Vitamin D3 data I have only found one estimate that says the average adult can make 20,000 IUs of D3 from just ½ hour of summer sunbathing in Finland at 62 degrees north. I have also seen musings by researchers claiming that after the skin has produced 20,000 IUs of D3 that the body might shut off further production-but they provide no evidence of this! I believe this is not true. Why? Because Israeli lifeguards have been found to have a 20X increased incidence of kidney stones as compared to the general Israeli population.

I one study form 1980 titled: Increased incidence of nephrolithiasis (kidney stones) in lifeguards in Israel. The researchers found that 11 of 45 (24%) of lifeguards had proven kidney stones. This is approximately 20X the incidence of kidney stones in the general population.

From the 1,000+ high dose Vitamin D3 self-experiments I have heard about; I have encountered three cases of kidney stones and those occurred in 3 people each taking about 50,000 IU per day of Vitamin D3 without Vitamin K2 after about a 6-month period. And one of the stone formers admitted it had run in his family as his brother had suffered kidney stones when he was in his 20's. Stones have been so rare in my 1,000+ sample set that I expect for 25% of the lifeguards to form kidney stones that they must have been making 100,000 to 200,000 or more of Vitamin D3 in their skin each day. The reason they were getting stones is that the high levels of D3 had depleted their K2 stores and thus the excess calcium went into their blood that was filtered out to become kidney stones. I have seen it repeated many times by leading Vitamin D researchers that Vitamin D toxicity (aka hypercalcemia) cannot occur from sunbathing because the body converts excess Vitamin D3 into inert components. I believe this lifeguard example shows that this is **not true**. There was also a recently reported case of Vitamin D toxicity in a man who sunbathed 6 to 8 hours a day for 2 weeks after he had been taking 10,000 IUs of D3 per day for 2.5 years with no problems. After the 2 weeks of intense sunbathing in southeast Asia excess calcium damaged his kidneys. There is no way 10,000 IU per day caused his problem; it had to be from his extreme sunbathing habits. Had he been taking Vitamin K2, he likely would have had no problems.

A Comprehensive Study of Sunbathing and Vitamin D3 Levels Is Essential to See What Evolution Provides as An Appropriate Dose D3 For Humans to Use Medicinally. It Is Obviously Much Higher Than What Is Considered "High Doses" By Current Mainstream Science.

Also, it should also be noted that not all sun is equal. When exposed to the same amount of UVB radiation, **a person who is 70 years old will make 75 percent less D3 than a 20-year-old** [source: Lee].

Patients with CYP24A1 mutations may be at an increased risk of Vitamin D toxicity, and clinicians can consider genetic testing if Vitamin D toxicity develops with doses less than 10 000 IU per day.

If you're fair skinned, sunburn easily and live in New York City, you would need to spend just four minutes outside on a sunny 4th of July to produce about 1,000 IU of Vitamin D, but that turns into 40 minutes on a sunny

New Year's Day. Under those same conditions, a person with dark skin would need 16 minutes on July 4 and about 4.5 hours on Jan. 1 to produce the same amount of D3.

Interesting Tidbits from:

A recent article titled Vitamin D Deficiency: An Important, Common, and Easily Treatable Cardiovascular Risk Factor? Came to some interesting conclusions which I summarize as follows:

Studies show people with obesity have significantly lower Vitamin D levels (less than 50%) compared to leaner individuals-possibly because D3 gets sequestered in the fat.

As you move north or south from the equator, Vitamin D levels drop, mirroring a rise in conditions like heart disease, diabetes, and high blood pressure. The connection is compelling.

A Finnish study of 10,000+ kids found that giving them 2,000 IU of Vitamin D daily in their first year dramatically reduced their risk (-78%!) of developing type 1 diabetes up to 31 years later.

Short-term UV exposure from tanning beds can temporarily boost Vitamin D and lower blood pressure. UVB radiation in a tanning bed 3 times per week for 3 months led to a 180% increase in 25(OH)D levels and a 6-mm Hg reduction in both systolic and diastolic pressures

Bad Reactions People Have Had to High Dose Vitamin D3

Magnesium Deficiency Symptoms-

I would say that maybe 5% or so of the 1,000+ people I have heard from who were conducting high dose Vitamin D3 self-experiments have had some bad reactions. The vast majority of these bad reactions have come when they first start dosing. And oddly, these rare bad reactions are for the most part **not caused by hypercalcemia** the dreaded boogeyman feared by doctors near and far. I would say about 90% of the bad reactions to high dose Vitamin D3 are **caused by magnesium deficiency also** known as hypomagnesia!

Why does high dose Vitamin D3 trigger magnesium deficiency symptoms in some people? Because the reactions that Vitamin D3 induces in your body also require large amounts of magnesium to be completed. **So, when you are taking high dose D3 you are eating up magnesium at a much faster rate than normal**.

From a 2019 study titled: Magnesium Supplementation in Vitamin D Deficiency.

The major points made were:
- Both Vitamin D and magnesium are crucial for overall health and disease prevention, but most adults lack enough of both.
- While Vitamin D deficiency is widely recognized and readily testable, **magnesium deficiency is widespread and goes unnoticed due to unreliable blood tests.** Vitamin D screening assay is readily available, but the reported lower limit of the normal range is **totally inadequate** for disease prevention.
- Mg and Vitamin D are used by all the organs in the body, and their deficiency states may lead to several chronic medical conditions, reversal of any of these conditions may not occur for several years after adequate replacement.
- Studies show adequate Vitamin D and magnesium can:
  - Reduce bone fractures and early death in older adults.
  - Lower the risk of Alzheimer's dementia.
- However, taking high doses of Vitamin D without supplementing magnesium can actually deplete your magnesium stores, worsening the problem!

The most common bad reactions to high dose Vitamin D3 are:

-Extreme Fatigue
-Insomnia
-Heart Rhythm Disturbances (Arrhythmias)
-Tachycardia (fast heart rate)
-Dizziness
-Falls
-Blood Pressure Changes
-Anxiety
-Panic Attacks
-Constipation

Less common:

-Hallucinations
-Confusion
-Weakness

As you will see in the magnesium section of this book, all of these "side effects" are not due to ingesting high dose D3; they are actually the result of high dose D3 aggravating an underlying severe magnesium deficiency. It is estimated that about 80% of us are magnesium deficient due to modern farming practices, and amongst the 80% there is a subset that is extremely deficient. It is these people who will have trouble when they first take high dose Vitamin D3.

Had anyone with these side effects had sufficient magnesium in their systems before taking D3 these side effects would never have materialized.

Let me share a few stories with you of cases I have heard about.

In Germany the most popular book about Vitamin D3 is titled Healthy in 7 Days. It is written by a Dr. who advocates everyone taking 100,000 IUs of Vitamin D3 per day for 7 days then dialing it back to a maintenance dose of 10,000 to 20,000 IUs per day. One day I received an email from a German man whose wife had tried this protocol and soon started having heart arrhythmias. They went to the emergency room and the doctors told the wife that she should have a pacemaker wire embedded in her heart to normalize her heart beats. They had not had the surgery when they emailed me. I told them… "NO DO NOT DO THIS! Stop the D3 and take large doses of magnesium until the heartbeat rhythm returns to normal. They heeded my advice and within a day or so her heart was back to normal, no pacemaker needed.

Next is the story of a female friend of my neighbor. She started taking 25,000 IU of D3 per day and was soon experiencing falls. So, she stopped the D3 and the falls stopped. I later heard that she had been drinking a somewhat large amount of liquor one night after trying to relax from some extremely stressful news. She started blacking out and falling down. This happened several times although she did not seem exceptionally drunk. She ended up in the hospital and **received a pacemaker for her heart**. (She probably would have been fine in an hour if they had given her a magnesium IV.) This was when a little light bulb went off in my head and I realized she had been falling down after taking 25,000 IU of D3 per day. I looked into it, and as I suspected, drinking alcohol; causes a dramatic loss of magnesium through your urine. This is especially interesting in that alcohol withdrawal from alcoholics causes delirium tremens as well as extreme magnesium deficiency. Both cases of her falls, from D3 and from alcohol, I believe were caused by extreme magnesium deficiency.

A doctor in Austria emailed me and said the high dose Vitamin D3 was making his heart beat too fast and he wanted to know what to do. I told him he was magnesium deficient and this was a symptom brought on by the D3 using up some of his magnesium. He injected himself with 1 gram of magnesium in solution and found that he got instant relief.

One lady taking high dose Vitamin D3 reported that one day she was going down an escalator, and at the bottom of the escalator she got dizzy and fell down. She was quite angry about it and blamed the Vitamin D3. She left a 1-star review for my book needless to say.

A large man, about 300 pounds+, was taking 20,000 IU per day of Vitamin D3 to try and cure his plantar fasciitis. It was working quite well, but after about 2 weeks of high dose D3 he had the first panic attack in his entire life which scared him so much he decided to quit taking Vitamin D3. Panic attacks are another symptom of magnesium deficiency.

Here was one of the scariest reactions to Vitamin D3 in a person's own words-

1.0 out of 5 stars <u>D3 regimen certainly not for everyone</u> July 16, 2015

I purchased this book approx. 1 1/2 years ago from Amazon. I totally believed it. I followed this Man's regimen and wound up in the hospital for a week where I was given multiple diagnoses including but not limited to cancer, diabetes and others. When the MD learned about the high doses of Vitamin D3 they ran new tests and I discontinued the D3, within a week I was no longer falling down and hallucinating. I had to close my office for a month. I can only say, this regimen is not for everyone. Certainly not for me.

I will now share with you a journal article that appeared in 2018 about a man, a nuclear physicist in England, who was taking somewhat high doses of Vitamin D3 for 2 years with no problem (60,000 IUs per day), He then had about a 4 week bout of diarrhea for some reason. Then all of the sudden one day he could not perform the simplest of tasks like operating a cassette tape player and was struck with extreme fatigue, and then constipation. The doctors, I believe, misdiagnosed him as having hypercalcemia ("Vitamin D toxicity") and treated him for that, when in fact he was most likely suffering from hypomagnesia! The article follows along with my comment to the article's author from whom I have received no response (the journal did suggest I write an article on hypomagnesia and submit it to them):

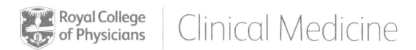

Clin Med (Lond). 2018 Aug; 18(4): 311–313.

Risks of the 'Sunshine pill' – a case of hypervitaminosis D

Case presentation

A 73-year-old man presented with a 4-week history of diarrhea and 2-week history of confusion. He was a retired nuclear scientist who was previously fully independent with no history of cognitive impairment. There was no history of smoking, alcohol or substance abuse.

His wife reported cognitive disturbances including being unable to use a cassette player or turn on his electric razor and he had started urinating in the sink. He was visited by his GP who found him confused, drowsy and dehydrated. Observations were unremarkable but a rectal examination showed hard stool in the rectum. Presuming a urinary tract infection, laxatives and trimethoprim were prescribed and he was transferred to hospital for further investigations.

On admission there were no infective signs or symptoms. His cardiovascular, respiratory and abdominal examinations were unremarkable. He was extremely delirious requiring sedation and occasional reasonable physical restraint. He scored 3/10 on the Abbreviated Mental Test Score (AMTS) but had no other neurological signs. His electrocardiogram (ECG), chest X-ray (CXR) and computed tomography (CT) brain were all normal. Admission blood test results are shown in Table Table1.

Table 1.

Patient's blood test results on admission (truncated to just abnormal results + magnesium).

Parameter	Results	Units	Normal
Hematocrit	0.375	L/L	0.38–0.54
Urea	9	mmol/L	2.5–7.8
Creatinine	202	umol/L	59–104
Procalcitonin	0.12	ng/mL	<0.25
Calcium	3.06	mmol/L	2.15–2.6
Corrected calcium	3.15	mmol/L	2.2–2.62
Magnesium	0.94	mmol/L	0.7–1
Ferritin	18	ug/L	22–322

Diagnosis

Investigations for his hypercalcemia revealed low parathyroid hormone 0.6 pmol/L and a toxic 25-hydroxyvitamin D (25[OH]D) concentration 881 nmol/L (normal range 25–100 nmol/L), ...

(my note this is 352 ng/ml compared to a US ref range of 30 to 100 ng/ml-this is high, but I have seen it this high before in others with no" toxic" effect. In fact, Vitamin D3 itself is completely nontoxic; it is simply information for your DNA - only the excess blood calcium or hypomagnesia can be dangerous)

…….. suggesting a diagnosis of hypervitaminosis D. Other causes of hypercalcemia such as malignancy, thyroid disease and sarcoidosis were excluded. On further questioning his daughter reported he had been taking 60,000 IU Vitamin D capsules per day for the last 2 years having read a book advocating its health benefits.

Initial management

According to **www.toxbase.org** guidelines, he was treated with intravenous fluids followed by a single dose of 60 mg pamidronate. Steroids were considered but not used in this case following discussion with endocrinology department colleagues.

Case progression and outcome

After 1 week of supportive treatment the patient showed signs of improvement with calcium concentrations and renal function now normal. His repeat AMTS was 6/10 as cognitively he started to recover. Two weeks after admission he was back to baseline and discharged home. Weekly blood tests were arranged over the next month to ensure no rebound hypercalcemia and all Vitamin D supplements were discontinued.

Discussion

Vitamin D is a fat-soluble vitamin essential for calcium homeostasis and bone health. Vitamin D2 (ergocalciferol) and D3 (cholecalciferol) can be obtained naturally from dietary sources (e.g. wild mushrooms and oily fish). Vitamin D3 is also formed by UV-B mediated conversion of 7-Dehydrocholesterol in the skin.[1] Due to a wide therapeutic index **hypervitaminosis D is extremely rare;** however, there are a small number of global case studies showing it can occur at excessively high doses of supplementation. The reported non-musculoskeletal health benefits of Vitamin D supplementation, including links to sepsis severity, acute respiratory distress syndrome (ARDS) and respiratory tract infections (RTIs) have seen its use increase significantly. There are also widespread claims in non-medical publications and the media that Vitamin D supplementation is a 'miracle cure'.

The right amount of Vitamin D

The Scientific Advisory Committee on Nutrition (SACN) and the National Institute for Health and Care Excellence (NICE) state that a 25(OH)D concentration below 30 nmol/L qualifies as Vitamin D deficient and there are clear links with poor musculoskeletal health. Apart from the possible prevention of RTIs, robust evidence linking Vitamin D deficiency to non-musculoskeletal diseases such as cancer, cardiovascular disease and obesity is still lacking. Autier *et al* suggest that low 25(OH)D concentrations may simply be a marker of ill health rather than primarily causing disease.

Conversely, Vitamin D toxicity with hypercalcemia can cause bone demineralization and both renal and cardiovascular toxicity.[12] The third National Health and Nutrition Examination Survey (NHANES III) also suggested that Vitamin D concentrations higher than 75 nmol/L could be associated with adverse effects, including increased mortality and incidence of cardiovascular disease.[15]

Based on the robust evidence for musculoskeletal outcomes alone, SACN and NICE currently recommend a Vitamin D reference nutrient intake (RNI) of 400 IU daily alongside sensible sun exposure for all healthy adults in the UK to prevent Vitamin D deficiency. Although there is currently no evidence for an optimal Vitamin D status, NICE states that serum 25(OH)D concentrations >50 nmol/L are 'adequate'. For Vitamin D deficient adults, the maximum dose for supplementation recommended by SACN should not exceed 4,000 IU/day. There are fixed loading regimes recommended by NICE, for example 50,000 IU once a week for 6 weeks (300,000 IU in total), and although these are not expected to cause adverse effects, may cause hypercalcemia in some individuals. 50,000 IU Vitamin D capsules are easily purchased on the internet and one has to question whether such high doses should be available to the public without prescription.

Pharmacokinetics and clinical course of hypervitaminosis D

To appreciate the clinical course of hypervitaminosis D, it is important to understand the pharmacokinetics. The lipophilic nature of Vitamin D explains its adipose tissue distribution. It has a slow turnover in the body with a half-life of approximately 2 months. Its main transport metabolite, 25(OH)D, has a half-life of 15 days while the more active metabolite, Calcitriol or 1,25(OH)2D, has a half-life of 15 hours. Therefore, depending on the level of toxicity, it can be expected that patients with hypervitaminosis D may exhibit symptoms for several weeks before showing signs of improvement.

Hypervitaminosis D treatment

The majority of symptoms are due to hypercalcemia; therefore, the mainstay of successful treatment in case reports has included initial rehydration with intravenous fluids followed by bisphosphonate therapy. Some cases were managed using diuretics, calcitonin or glucocorticoids as second line treatment. We consulted Toxbase and local endocrinology expertise to guide treatment. Due to the risk of rebound hypercalcemia and arrhythmias, we monitored biochemical parameters and ECGs regularly. **Given the fact that hypervitaminosis D is so rare** it is important to also consider and exclude other causes of hypercalcemia during treatment.

Key learning points

- Hypervitaminosis D is **a rare condition** and can be life-threatening
- (my note-this was actually a case of severe magnesium deficiency)

131

- Given the increasing self-supplementation and medical prescriptions of Vitamin D, consider hypervitaminosis D as a differential diagnosis in patients presenting with hypercalcemia *(my note-his blood calcium was high but not extraordinarily high-hypercalcemia was the wrong diagnosis)*
- Refer to the SACN and NICE guidelines for Vitamin D intake and supplementation in adults to prevent and treat Vitamin D deficiency
- Important for clinicians to understand the pharmacokinetics of Vitamin D to help predict the clinical course of patients with hypervitaminosis D
- The mainstay of hypervitaminosis D treatment involves the correction of hypercalcemia with rehydration and bisphosphonate therapy.

End article, Article link>
https://academic.oup.com/jn/article/134/6/1299/4688802

My Response to the Journal and the lead author

Hello Dr. Ellis-
I read your interesting article and noticed the patient had read a book on high dose Vitamin D3- I am probably the author. I would like to explain to you what you were probably

looking at. The elevated calcium on his test was likely not the culprit as it was just moderately elevated compared to the reference range. What you were witnessing was magnesium deficiency symptoms, as high dose Vitamin D3 will burn up a lot of magnesium, and most of us are magnesium deficient to begin with. Amongst magnesium deficiency symptoms are included: confusion (long term symptom), as well as constipation, and fatigue. It was also noted that the patient had chronic diarrhea for several weeks which could have reduced his magnesium levels even further. The blood tests for magnesium are highly unreliable as only 1% of the body's magnesium is found in blood and it is tightly controlled. His magnesium should have been tested with the oral load test or a muscle biopsy. So. his "normal" magnesium score likely hid a major magnesium deficiency in his tissues-exacerbated by 2 years of high dose Vitamin D3 use. He could have been quickly treated with a magnesium IV and he probably would have been perfectly fine in an hour. And then you should have educated him on the requirement to co-supplement with magnesium while taking high doses of Vitamin D3.

If he was being affected by hypercalcemia his calcium levels would likely have been much higher, and the first symptoms are loss of appetite, nausea, vomiting, and rapid weight loss, and/or kidney stones/kidney failure. Your report did not mention any of these hypercalcemia symptoms, **so it is much more likely a case of Vitamin D3 and diarrhea induced hypomagnesia.** Any thoughts? Jeff T. Bowles

The bottom-line learning point I take away from the prior examples of magnesium deficiency symptoms are that they are not to be ignored, minimized, or trifled with! It has become evident that the symptoms can be very dangerous for the few unlucky people who start high dose Vitamin D3 from a magnesium deficient state. While Vitamin D3 induced magnesium deficiency symptoms are rather rare. What is even more rare is the big bugaboo that doctors fear so much for almost no reason- hypercalcemia or excess calcium in the blood.

Bad Reactions People Have Had to High Dose Vitamin D3

Hypercalcemia Symptoms-

I have heard about at least 1,000 high dose Vitamin D3 experiments, likely many more. And one thing I have rarely seen is anyone experiencing hypercalcemia. I can count on one hand the number of cases and I will discuss them here. From my point of view the cases of hypercalcemia occur in about ½ of 1% of the cases of high dose Vitamin D3 supplementation and **all of those were likely preventable** with Vitamin K2 supplements. In fact, I know of one man who takes 1 million IUs per day with lots of Vitamin K2 for his MS and has been doing so for more than a year now. All the while his blood calcium remains in the low normal range! See the case of Zoran Vujicic in the MS article you read earlier.

The first three cases I heard about were people who developed calcium kidney stones from taking high dose Vitamin D3. The first two cases were quite similar. Both people had read my book. One was a man in his 50's and the other a younger lady, both developed kidney stones after about 5 to 6 months of supplementing with about 50,000 IU of Vitamin D3 per day. In both cases they admitted to not taking the amount of Vitamin K2 suggested in the book. The man had taken just one super K pill with his 50,000 a day when he should have been taking at least 5 and maybe 10 Super K pills. (Super K pills contain 200mcg of the MK7 type of K2 and

1000 mcg of the MK4 type of K2). The man admitted that kidney stones ran in his family and that his brother had gotten one in his 20's.

The lady decided to get her Vitamin K2 by eating ghee (similar to butter) made from grass-fed cow's milk. The lady had suffered some bad effects when she first started her high dose D3 such as insomnia and fatigue but those were ameliorated when she started taking larger doses of magnesium.

After they passed their kidney stones, they had no other negative effects. And they both started taking more Vitamin K2 with their D3.

There was a third lady who claimed to have been giving 50,000 IU of Vitamin D per day from her doctors with no Vitamin K2 she had not read my book but just left a comment in the review section and claimed to have developed a severe case of kidney stones that required multiple surgeries to correct. She might have been prescribed Vitamin D2 which is more likely to cause hypercalcemia than D3-this point was not clear. In her own words:

"It was a calcium blockage the size of a grape tomato and it was at the ureter, which was extremely dangerous as voiding completely was not happening but being blocked and I had no knowledge except as I said, something did not seem right. They first had to put a stent in, but they were unable to do so given the size and location, so I had to have an extremely painful and humiliating procedure done in which an invasive operation from the back which included a catheter which went to my leg. As a woman especially, this was very upsetting, and I had to have this in me for months, and at times, had infections. It also ended up having to be removed as it was wrapped around my bladder, and that was before the next 4 surgeries to destroy the blockage. I finally found a wonderful surgeon who, had I gone to him in the beginning, I would probably never have had to have that awful catheter. My heart goes out to people who need that on a permanent basis.

I did not take K2, but I am not sure it would have prevented this, but who knows? I agree about our medical world and after this experience, I will always do my homework before any recommendations again. "

So that was it for kidney stones. The takeaway? Skimp on Vitamin K2 at your own risk!

Now there were 2 cases of hypercalcemia that I heard about. In both cases I was contacted by the wife of a man who had developed hypercalcemia. And one of the men had read my book the other hadn't.

Case #1-A man had heard from a nurse that taking Vitamin D3 was good for you. So, on his own he decided to take approximately 300,000 IU of Vitamin D3 per day without any Vitamin K2 (he apparently did not know about K2). All was fine for a while, several months, and then according to his wife he started feeling nauseous, was throwing up and was rapidly losing weight. (These are all classic signs of hypercalcemia and he should have stopped the D3 at these first signs). The man figured that he simply had a stomach bug and kept on taking the 300,000 IU of D3 per day! He lost about 40 pounds in 6 weeks. From 180 to 140! He got sick enough to end up in the emergency room, and he was admitted to the hospital with borderline kidney failure! He was put on an IV to dilute the calcium out of his blood and kidneys and given other meds. After two weeks he was released, and he eventually got back to normal after a month or so. I sent his wife a free copy of my D3 book after this incident!

Case #2 A man's wife was searching for a cure for his ankylosing spondylitis, a terrible form of arthritis that eventually often leads to severe curvature of the spine. She apparently had read my book and told him to try high dose Vitamin D3. He supposedly got excellent results right off the bat at 25,000 IU per day. It alleviated almost all of his pain. But supposedly the pain would come back little by little so he would up the dose, and the pain was at bay again. He got into this cycle and upped his dose over and over and eventually was taking 600,000 IU per day with almost no Vitamin K2. Maybe one super K pill per day. Well, after about 9 months after he started, he ended up in the emergency room unable to eat, vomiting and experiencing rapid weight loss. Again, the classic signs of hypercalcemia. The doctors told him to stop the D3 which he did and wait for his blood D3 and calcium levels to return back to normal in a month or two. All well and good except in his case he started experiencing the most extreme pain he could imagine throughout his bones! He was taking supposedly up to 20 Oxycontin a day to try and stop the pain but nothing worked. I remembered, based on my self-experimentation, that melatonin seemed to counteract the effects of Vitamin D3 in some areas, so I suggested they experiment with high dose melatonin to counteract the D3 induced pain. Luckily it worked and he was able to drop his oxycontin intake to just 1 a day until his D3 levels finally got back to normal. The wife later told me she finally found a cure for ankylosing spondylitis through the use of higher doses of boron-more on this later.

In all but one of these cases of hypercalcemia it is good to know that there was no long-term damage or irreversible side effects like the kind you can get with Big Pharma's drugs!

So that's it; those are all the negative experiences in more than 1,000+ high dose Vitamin D3 experiments I have directly heard about. Not so bad. All of them seemed easily preventable with a little foresight and intelligent co-supplementation.

Are Some Vitamin D Researchers Intentionally Sabotaging Their Experiments to Discourage the Use of Vitamin D3?

I recently did a several weeks long research project to get to the bottom of the question- what do researchers consider "high dose" when experimenting with Vitamin D3? I went to the PubMed medical study database to see what most researchers considered "high dose" when conducting a Vitamin D3 study.

What I found was both exhilarating and disturbing!

You can do the same research yourself- just go to google, search the term PubMed, then log into their database and search the following terms. Type it exactly as shown>

"high dose Vitamin D3" OR "high-dose Vitamin D"

There were 407 results out of about 82,000 total abstracts that now mention Vitamin D since 1922. The number of abstracts from this search will grow a bit as more studies are added, at the date of this writing (10/2019) it has grown to 412.

I only reviewed what was written in the abstract and did not dig any further to read the actual journal article.

In 130 of the studies Vitamin D3 was found to effectively treat the studied issue or disease while 112 studies found Vitamin D3 ineffective. 165

studies did not say whether there was a particular outcome.

I designated 39 studies as "WOW" studies that had some particularly impressive results.

Here were my notes for the "WOW" studies with the daily dose indicated where reported in the abstract:

Helps autism symptoms
For kidney disease in diabetics 10k/d
Food allergies in kids

HighdoseD3 + omega 3 HALTS TYPE 1 diab
  preserved beta cells
Autistic kids 5k/day

D3 for gut micro flora in Cystic fibrosis
Incrs Huntington's life from 73 to 101 days

Stops/reverses pancreatic cancer! 50k/d
1 x dose for diabetic neuropathy

CURES ichthyosis!! 60k/day
to incr D3 in infants YES SAFE
Cured 14/16 psoriasis vitiligo!
35,000/day
High dose D3 helps ALS
Cured immun thrombo cytopenia in elderly

Internet search cites 37 **cures** of IBS

1 case WORKED for MS

COPD cure
1x dose for cyst fibrosis lung
Spont.Osteonecrosisknee decrPain
Fibromyalgia!
Treats reactive airway dysfunction
Sickle cell anemia pain 100% GONE!
2000/day to infants=>taller kids!!!
MS

For Back and hip pain!

INFANTS   FLU STOPS IT (like
12,000 day)
Cures HIVES!!
IBD CURED!!!
Haily blistering disease CURED
D3&mg
High dose D3 +Omg-3 >Type1
Diabetes in remission

CURES myasthenia gravis!! 120k/day
Decr HIV replication in aids!!!
D3 very low in cystic fibrosis patients
Vitamin D3 to prevent all diseases
give moms D3>decr TYPE 1 diabetes
risk in kids!

143

RDA way too low incr D3 to stop diseases!
50k vit d2 + calcium>>hypercalcemia
40k d3/day ok
D3 increases risk of falls 3X in nursing
homes
**So, amongst these 39 "wow" studies my favorites
are-**

-Type I diabetes which occurs in children can be
halted in its tracks with high dose Vitamin D3 and
fish oil., and then there is no need for increasing
insulin doses because the disease no longer
progresses!

-An 83 year old woman with terminal pancreatic
cancer was sent home to die but unbeknownst to
her doctors she had been and continued to take
50,000 IUs of D3 per day; after 8 months they
were surprised she was still alive, reexamined her
and found that her pancreatic tumor was shrinking.
The woman said she never felt better!

--35,000 IUs /day of D3 cured 14 / 16 psoriasis and
vitiligo cases. The remaining two uncured patients
probably needed higher doses.

-Myasthenia Gravis went into complete remission
for the first time in a woman taking 80,000 to
120,000 IUs of D3 per day.

Okay so much for the exhilarating stuff. What did I find so disturbing? I marked some studies with the word "bias" when it looked to me like the investigators were intentionally using too low a dose of D3 to have any effect, were rigging the experiment to fail, or were making negative comments about Vitamin D3.

Of the 292 studies that listed the dose of D3 given to study participants in the abstract only 37 used daily (equivalent) doses of 10,000 IU per day or more. While 41 studies used 2,000 IU per day or less! In other words, high dose Vitamin D3 supplementation has barely been studied!

Here are the studies where D3 was described as having no benefit or being harmful:

D3 increases infections!   Univ Wisc 2017
CVD didn't work   Harvard   2019
MS   Norway   2019 3k/day
pneumonia x-ray New Zealand   2018 5k/day
no decr adverse events Harvard nz   2018 3k/day
10k/kg/day!! Colitis Australia   2018
D3 2prevent cancer Harvard   2018 3k/day
2help knee replacemenHarvard   2018 2k/day
VITAL ongoing HARVARD!!!   2018 2k/day
4k day obese blacks Harvard duke   2015 4k/day
type 2 diabetes Canada   2012 2k/day
diabetes Korea   2015 2k/day
 5500/d 6 wks typ2 diabetesDenmark 2015 5k/day

for BP 200k/mo.42 mos.New Zealand 2015
diabetes 511 Norway   2014
1 x /year no help depression   2012
Hypercalc in MS patient ppmsAustria 2019 5k/day
no benefit HIGH RISKNew Zealand 2018
HYPERcalcemia granulomatous   2017 8k/day
"high dose D3 does not work in MS" 2013
"d3 4 UC reduce bone density!"no K2 2013
20 to 40/week for cholesterol   2013 6k/day
"incr D3 increases fracture!"   2013
puppy injected w D3 calcified!   2004
D3 + cancer   2019
D3 + cancer   Harvard new zlnd 2019
no help mentalillnessHarvrd Tufts   2019 2k/day
"high dose"1,000 IUs / day   Canada   2015 1k/day
for MS 5k vs 600 /dayYale UCLA   2015 5k/day
"lowest dose 2cause "hypercalc"   2008 4k/day
400 iu/kg/day 4 liver damage Turkey 2018
hypercalc kids!Turkey from ca >10.5! 2019
kids w/osteogenesis imperfecta   2016 2k/day
"no effect gene express!!!Oxford   2018 4k/day

(Before I get started, if anyone would like a copy of
the excel spread sheet I created with this data please
send me an email at Jeffbo at aol dot com and
I'll happily send it right over.)

The disturbing thing I saw in a lot of these studies I
believed to be biased against Vitamin D3 is the
huge involvement of Harvard in cranking out these

studies. Harvard has been putting out study after study saying Vitamin D3 has no effect on this or that, lending its supposed authoritative name to absolute JUNK SCIENCE meant to, I believe, discourage everyone from using Vitamin D3 for therapeutic purposes. 2,000 IUs per day is what Harvard runs most of its studies with which is not enough to do much of anything other than to prevent colds. 2,000 IUs is equivalent to about 3 minutes of sunbathing per day. It is a real scandal. And these studies they are doing are HUGE, they cover many years and have more than 20,000 participants in many cases! (Google the VITAL studies) Also the universities in the countries of New Zealand, Norway, and Turkey also all seem to be in on this disinformation campaign. And if you add any institutions doing studies of "high dose" D3 with 2000 IUs you could include institutions in Finland and Denmark to the culprit list as well. And it seems that a lot of these low dose studies are coming out in a big way since 2018 and 2019! They are right in the middle of the disinformation campaign as we speak!

I would also like to add Google as being in on this disinformation campaign. A few years ago, when I started my website JeffTbowles.com, I wrote and published article after article showing how high dose Vitamin D3 cured this or that disease complete with multiple self-reported case studies for each. In the beginning all was fine and most of my articles would appear within the first 4 pages in search results (and usually on page 1) when you Googled a disease and the term "cure" and "Vitamin D3". But some time in 2019, Google changed its rating of my site to make sure none of my articles were found easily. For example, my #1 article the Overwhelming Proof that Vitamin D3 Deficiency Causes Most Human Diseases used to show up on page 1 in the #1 or #2 slot when anyone searched "Vitamin D3" and "latitude" on Google. One day it was just gone. They deep-sixed it with no explanation. Now you can search "Vitamin D3" and "latitude" and you cannot find my article anywhere in the first 40 pages-I haven't searched past 40 on Google but it shows up on page 1 of all the other search engines. Also, I used to get about 90% of my search traffic from Google, and that has fallen to about 50%, and sometimes as low as 33%. Luckily my traffic from the other legitimate search engines has been increasing to offset Google's sabotage of alternative health information websites.

Now this did not just happen to me but also to a great website run by Dr Mercola. He had a lot of fantastic articles about alternative medicine. Some were a little sketchy but overall his site was overwhelmingly helpful and hugely popular. One day if you searched Google for information that appeared on Mercola's site. Nothing! He was gone;

his search hits from Google decreased by 99% from maybe millions a day, overnight!

I believe google has been infiltrated and corrupted by some Big Pharma and AMA moles to try to suppress this life-saving information from getting to you. Harvard and Google! What ever happened to first do no harm!????

From the Perrymarshall dot com's website:

- Google no longer cares what people are looking for...they're more interested in TELLING people what they are looking for
- Why Google's new quality rater guidelines are a death knell for experts whose views threaten industry profits
- Why Google now buries expert views if they're deemed "harmful" to the public...and the dubious process they use to determine "harmful"
- Why even board-certified experts like Dr. Mercola, (whose articles are fully referenced, most containing dozens of references to studies published in the peer-reviewed scientific literature) get canceled when their views contradict the industries cozy with Google
- How Google's previously "democratic system" has now morphed into "let's grab all

the power we can by forcing our partners'
beliefs on the manipulated masses"

If anyone wants to search for health information, I
suggest they use only **Bing**, Yahoo or Duckduckgo.
Google is corrupted when it comes to health care
information and is no longer your friend, they now
seem to be in the pocket of Big Pharma and the
AMA to help continue the golden gravy train for
Big Pharma and mainstream medicine. They do not
want you to see this information.

Magnesium Deficiency-

I estimate that magnesium deficiency causes up to about 20% of all human disease, from heart and blood pressure disturbances to neurological/mental problems and much more. (Refer to the list of symptoms of magnesium deficiency later in this chapter.)

Estimates of how many people are magnesium deficient in industrialized countries range as high as 88%!

Why don't doctors know this or test for this? Because the adult human body contains about 25 grams of magnesium, 60% in the bones and about 40% in the soft tissues. Only 1% is found in the blood and it is tightly regulated. Anytime you need more blood magnesium it is taken from the bones or soft tissues and the blood level remains relatively constant. If the blood magnesium gets out of whack just a little bit you will immediately know it due to fainting, dizziness, falls, panic attacks, abnormal heart rhythms, heart palpitations, large blood pressure changes, cramps, and many more-see below

Because blood magnesium is tightly controlled, there is no good or easy blood test for magnesium deficiency. So **almost no doctor knows the level of magnesium in your body.** There are more difficult tests like "inject and collect" which means

151

you get a large injection of magnesium solution and then you have to collect your urine for 24 hours and see how much magnesium flows through with your urine. If nothing comes out in your urine, you are very magnesium deficient! I bet almost anyone reading this has never had this test. That is why **80%+ of us can be magnesium deficient and the doctors have no clue!**

The most practical way to determine if you are magnesium deficient is to look at the long list of symptoms and if you have one some or many of them it points towards magnesium deficiency. Many people taking a daily magnesium supplement may still be magnesium deficient as it is a very difficult deficiency to correct! Also, the older you are the harder it is to absorb magnesium and thus the elderly are at more risk of magnesium deficiency diseases than younger demographics.

How did we all become so magnesium deficient? "Modern" farming practices that are designed to grow big healthy-looking fruits and vegetables quickly without regard to their nutritional content have caused almost all foods produced today to be very low in magnesium compared to times past.

According to nutrition experts, the magnesium content of foods has been declining dramatically since preindustrial times and continues at an accelerated rate. In 2004, the Journal of the

American College of Nutrition released a study which compared nutrient content of crops at that time with 1950 levels. Declines were found as high as 40%.

Dr. Donald Davis, who conducted the study, describes the last 50 years in farming as being a period where farmers were looking for new varieties of fruits, crops and vegetables that provide pest resistance, higher yields, and greater flexibility in what climates they can be grown in. But the main push was for higher yields which leads to crops that grow big very quickly which reduces the amount of nutrients they can absorb from the soil.

Just looking at the food tables from the USDA in the US and the Food Standards Agency in the UK you find large declines in magnesium up until the 1990's and it has only gotten worse since then:

Magnesium Content-	Percentage Decline U.S. 1963 – 1992
Avg. decline for fruits & vegetables studied	21%
Spinach	10%
Corn	23%
Carrots	35%
Collard Greens	84%

Declines in magnesium affects more than just fruits and vegetables. A study in Nutrition and

Health examined average nutritional content of foods across food categories in the UK:

From 1940 to 1991 magnesium in-

Vegetables declined by 24%

- Fruit declined by   17%.
- Meat declined by   15%.
- Cheeses declined by 26%.

And these are old studies – the decline in magnesium continues to this day!

In addition to reduced absorption of magnesium by plants, another major probable cause of widespread magnesium deficiency is the declining magnesium content of soils around the modern world. This is caused by using fertilizers as a substitute for the traditional practice of crop rotation. Thus, you get the same crop every year from the same land, taking specific minerals like magnesium out of the soil year after year. And because farm fertilizers are not regulated for required additives, farmers simply choose the cheapest fertilizers without regard to mineral content.

For example, many farmers use the potassium fertilizer potash which is easily, and quickly absorbed by plants, but this reduces the amount of magnesium and calcium absorbed. Modern nitrogen fertilizers give us bigger produce, but with fewer nutrients.

Agricultural expert Charles Benbrook, Ph.D., recently explained the phenomenon:

"High nitrogen levels make plants grow fast and bulk up with carbohydrates and water. While the fruits these plants produce may be big, they suffer in nutritional quality. The farmers prosper under this system, but the consumer suffers by paying more for bigger, better looking but vitamin and mineral deficient produce."

So, the final conclusion we can take away from all this is-

YOU CANNOT GET ENOUGH MAGNESIUM FROM

A MODERN DIET ALONE!

EVERYONE MUST SUPPLEMENT WITH MAGNESIUM EVERYDAY!

What happens when you are magnesium deficient?

Magnesium Deficiency Symptoms and Diseases

A magnesium deficiency can affect virtually every system of the body.

Early signs-
-Leg cramps

155

-Foot pain
-Muscle twitching
-Constipation
-Fatigue-extreme
-Weakness
-Insomnia
-Numbness
-Tingles
-Personality changes (Mag deficient people may seem tense)
-Abnormal heart rhythms
-Panic attacks
-Heart palpitations
-Heart arrhythmias
-Fainting, dizziness, & falls (vertigo)
-High blood pressure
-Large blood pressure changes
-Angina due to coronary artery spasms
-Coronary spasms

Longer Term Symptoms of Magnesium Deficiency-
-Type II (adult onset) diabetes
-Muscle tension/soreness,
-Back pain
-Neck pain
-Tension headaches
-Migraine headaches
-TMJ (jaw joint dysfunction)
-Chest tightness

-Frozen Shoulder (see my story at the end of the boron chapter)
-Tendonitis
-Calcifications
-Loss of appetite (similar to hypercalcemia symptoms)
-Nausea (similar to hypercalcemia symptoms)
-Vomiting (similar to hypercalcemia symptoms)
-Breathing difficulties -as if you can't breathe deeply
-Sighing a lot
-Chronic fatigue syndrome (my addition)
-Hypertension
-Hypothyroidism (Your body needs iodine & magnesium to make T4)
-Depressed immune response
-Urinary spasms
-Menstrual cramps
-Swallowing difficulty
-Lump in the throat-often caused by consuming sugar
-Odd sensations, buzzes, nerve vibrations
-Salt craving
-Swelling of legs and ankles after sitting long periods
-Carbohydrate craving especially chocolate
-Carbohydrate intolerance
-Poor digestion
-Breast tenderness
-Tinnitus (ringing in the ears)

-Cataracts
-Hearing loss
-Atrial Fibrillation
-Heart failure
-Myocardial infarction
-Sudden cardiac death
-Stroke

Mental Issues Caused by Magnesium Deficiency-
-Photophobia (hard to adjust to bright lights)
-Noise sensitivity
-Anxiety
-Insomnia
-Panic attacks
-Personality changes (Mag deficient people appear tense)
-Hyperactivity /restlessness / constant movement
-Irritability
-Hypothyroidism (magnesium required to make T4)
-Agoraphobia (fear of places/situations that might cause you to panic)
-Premenstrual irritability (PMS)
-Hyperexcitable
-Apprehensive
-Belligerent
-Clouded thinking
-Psychotic behavior
-Confusion
-Disorientation
-Depression

-Terrifying hallucinations from delirium tremens
-Tantrums (consider if increasing magnesium deficiency in the population as a possible cause of mental changes that lead to mass shootings?)

Long Term Skeletal Consequences of Magnesium Deficiency
-Calcification of organs
-Tooth decay
-Poor bone development
-Osteoporosis
-Slow healing of broken or fractured bones

Extreme Consequences of Magnesium Deficiency-
-Seizures,
-Mitral valve prolapse
-Cachexia & Death (more on this shortly)
Be aware that not all of the symptoms need to be present to be diagnosed with a magnesium deficiency; but many often occur together. For example, people with mitral valve prolapse frequently have palpitations, arrhythmias, anxiety, PMS, and panic attacks. Magnesium deficient people usually seem tense.

And When Blood Levels Get Too Low

(Remember these when we examined High Dose Vitamin D3 induced magnesium deficiency symptoms?)

****Although rare, in general, these are the magnesium deficiency symptoms I have heard about **most frequently when some people start taking high dose Vitamin D3**.****

-Fainting
-Dizziness
-Falls
-Abnormal heart rhythm
-Insomnia
-Panic attacks
-Palpitations
-Heart arrhythmias
-Extreme fatigue
-Insomnia
-Blood pressure changes

And in **rare cases**- extreme confusion or hallucinations.

Every cell in your body requires magnesium to function. It is involved in hundreds of reactions involving the cell. It is also required in the production of proteins, and for the use of sugars and fats for energy. Magnesium is also essential for detoxification reactions. Magnesium deficiency affects every cell in your body in a very negative way. Doctors prescribe tranquilizers to millions every year simply to treat symptoms of magnesium deficiency such as anxiety, irritability, and unease.

The brain is highly affected by magnesium deficiency.

Anxiety, anger, panic attacks, confusion, irritability, tantrums, and even terrifying hallucinations can be caused by magnesium deficiency.

(Could the increasing scourge of mass shootings plaguing the US be related to increasing rates of magnesium deficiency amongst the population? I think a great study would be to determine the magnesium content of tissue samples from mass shooters).

Calcium is lost in the urine while magnesium deficient; this lack of magnesium can cause osteoporosis, tooth decay, bone synthesis problems, and impaired healing of fractures and breaks.

When taken with Vitamin B6 (pyridoxine), magnesium helps to dissolve calcium kidney stones.

It is quite likely that **magnesium deficiency is the main cause of atrial fibrillation**. In one Canadian study it was found that intravenous magnesium corrected patients' heart rhythms in 84% of the cases.

The Extreme Difficulty of Reversing a Magnesium Deficiency-

161

Most people assume that if they are magnesium deficient that they can simply take a daily magnesium supplement and reverse the deficiency. This is not true in many cases.

Because 99% of your magnesium is located in your bones and soft tissues, and magnesium supplements enter your blood then leave through your urine. It can take a long, long time to reverse the magnesium deficits in your bones and soft tissues. In fact, Dr, Carolyn Dean the author of the Magnesium Miracle notes that it can take **a YEAR OR MORE** to build up the magnesium content of your bone and muscles (which includes your heart).

An article titled "Subclinical magnesium deficiency: a principal driver of cardiovascular disease and a public health crisis can be summarized as follows:

- Magnesium deficiency can be hiding in plain sight!
- Most magnesium (99%) lives inside cells, not in your blood. That's why normal blood levels often mask a hidden deficiency lurking within.
- Modern life is a magnesium thief; chronic diseases, medications, and processed foods can deplete your stores.

- Magnesium is a powerhouse; over 300 enzymes that operate in your bones, muscles, brain, heart, and more rely on it.
- Magnesium deficiency leads to osteoporosis, mental issues, heart problems, and many chronic conditions.
- A "normal" blood test doesn't guarantee healthy magnesium levels. In fact, most of them are worthless. Your body can steal from bones and muscles to keep blood levels up, masking a deeper deficiency.

One expert has argued that a typical Western diet may provide enough magnesium to avoid an **obvious** magnesium deficiency, but it is unlikely to maintain high enough magnesium levels to reduce the risk of the long list of magnesium deficiency associated diseases. Studies have shown that at least 300 mg magnesium must be supplemented to establish significantly increased serum magnesium to lower their risk of developing many chronic diseases. **So, while the recommended daily allowance (RDA) for magnesium (between 300 and 420 mg/day for most people) may prevent obvious magnesium deficiency, it is unlikely to prevent long term chronic conditions or deadly diseases.**

For example, among apparently healthy university students in Brazil, 42% were found to have magnesium deficiency. The average

163

magnesium intake was only around 215 mg/day.

Doctors use reference ranges to determine what is "normal" for various nutrients, hormones and vitamins. The assumption behind using these reference ranges is that the overall population has a healthy amount of substance in their blood on average. In the case of magnesium this is just not true. In fact, up to 88% of the population is now believed to be magnesium deficient. So, when your doctor shows you that you have a "normal" blood magnesium level, yes you do- but you are still bone and tissue-deficient just like almost everyone else!! If your blood magnesium is low according to the doctor's tests -look out! That means you are almost certainly very deficient in your tissues. Also, the blood test is a barely reliable guide at all! The magnesium content of the plasma is an unreliable guide to body stores: muscle is a more accurate guide to the body content of magnesium. If you want a truly accurate test of your magnesium levels – get a muscle biopsy- ouch!

Another study highlighting the discrepancy between serum and body magnesium levels concluded: 'Although blood-K (K here = potassium) and blood-Mg values in patients receiving long-term treatment for hypertension or heart disease usually are normal, **muscle-Mg and muscle-K are deficient in about 50% of these patients.**

If you really want an accurate idea of the magnesium levels in your body, the muscle biopsy method is fast and accurate. Another way to test for Mg deficiency is the inject magnesium and collect the urine for 24 hours. No magnesium excretion = deficiency.

Another more accurate test for Magnesium deficiency is the oral load test. In a 1993 study titled-
The oral magnesium loading test for detecting possible magnesium deficiency.
The key points were:

- Standard blood tests usually miss magnesium deficiency.
- The Oral Magnesium Load Test (OMLT) offers a promising solution.
  - Athletes take a dose of magnesium lactate (5g) and their urine is tested.
  - Low magnesium excretion suggests deficiency, even with normal blood levels.
- In a study of top athletes, 42% showed deficiency on the OMLT, despite normal blood tests.

- Ten days of magnesium supplementation improved absorption and reduced deficiency in some athletes.

Another study found that 10 out of 11 apparently healthy women were magnesium-deficient based on the oral magnesium load test.

The most dramatic change that has occurred since the early 1900s until now regarding phosphate, calcium and magnesium in foods **has been a reduction in magnesium intake, going from around 500 mg/day to an average of 250 mg/day**

The prevalence and incidence of type 2 diabetes in the United States increased sharply between 1994 and 2001. One study noticed a 3.25X increased risk of diabetes when plasma magnesium levels <0.863 mmol/L (despite 0.75 mmol/L being considered a 'normal' level). Thus, **magnesium deficiency likely increases the risk of diabetes and may even be its cause. Although low D3 levels have been implicated as well. Type II diabetes is likely caused by the one-two punch of low D3 and magnesium levels.**

Dietary aluminum may also lead to a magnesium deficit by reducing the absorption of magnesium by approximately 80%, reducing magnesium retention by 40% and causing less magnesium to be deposited in the bone. Aluminum is everywhere in society such as in tea, spinach, aluminum pots and pans, various medications, deodorant, baking powder, processed cheeses, potatoes, etc.

A Vitamin B 6-deficient diet can also lead to a magnesium deficiency due to increased magnesium excretion.

Another study found that young women may be losing magnesium despite consuming 350 mg of magnesium per day. Other data have found negative magnesium balance in men with osteoporosis or mental illness consuming 240 mg/day of magnesium. Another study noted negative magnesium balance (−122 mg) in those consuming 322 mg/day of magnesium with a high-fiber diet.

Older people are at higher risk of magnesium deficiency due to low intake and also due to having higher rates of diseases that exacerbate magnesium deficiency. **Aging also reduces magnesium absorption in the gut**.

A 1994 review article titled- Magnesium metabolism and perturbations in the elderly can be summarized with these key pints:

The elderly are at higher risk of magnesum deficiency: magnesium deficiency.

- Dietary changes and picky eating habits often leave seniors short on magnesium.

- Intestinal Absorption slowdown in aging bodies lead to a struggle to soak up this crucial mineral from food.

- Increased urinary output depletes magnesium stores further.

- Magnesium inhibits pathological calcification, and a deficiency can contribute to formation of calcium kidney stones.

- The result? Many older adults suffer from magnesium deficiency, putting them at risk for heart problems, kidney stones, and brittle bones.

Magnesium deficiency-Causes

Numerous factors can lead to magnesium deficiency, such as kidney failure, alcohol consumption and absorption issues (magnesium is absorbed in the small intestine and in the colon, thus, patients with intestinal or colon damage such as Crohn's disease, irritable bowel syndrome, celiac disease, gastroenteritis, ulcerative colitis, resection of the small intestine, ileostomy may have magnesium deficiency). Renal tubular acidosis, diabetic acidosis, prolonged diuresis, acute pancreatitis, hyperparathyroidism and primary aldosteronism can also lead to magnesium deficiency. A review of 5500 patients found that magnesium levels were significantly lower in patients with metabolic syndrome versus controls. The intravenous magnesium tolerance test showed that children with type 1 diabetes have intracellular magnesium deficiency.

Supplementing with calcium can lead to magnesium deficiency due to competitive inhibition for absorption, and over supplementing with Vitamin D may lead to magnesium deficiency via excessive calcium absorption which increases the risk of arterial calcification. (This risk can be reduced or eliminated with concomitant supplementation of large doses of Vitamin K2 and magnesium). Use of diuretics and other medications can also lead to magnesium deficiency.

Magnesium Deficiency-Related Cachexia:

What is cachexia? It is defined as ... the weakness and wasting of the body due to severe chronic illness. Some call it the final illness.

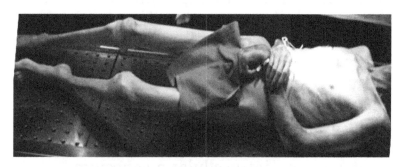

You probably know what it is if I describe it as you see it in real life. Have you ever had a relative who was dying of cancer or old age? When they are getting towards the end, they just lose the desire to eat, and just start losing weight no matter what treatment you give them to try and stimulate their appetite Eventually they just waste away to nothing. This happens as well to people with various chronic diseases that become terminal. Doctors have tried many things to boost the appetite: medical marijuana, appetite stimulants, thalidomide, cytokine inhibitors, steroids, nonsteroidal anti-inflammatory drugs, branched-chain amino acids, eicosapentaenoic acid (EPA), and ant serotoninergic drugs.

Nothing has worked very well; progesterone has helped some, but about 50% of cancer patients actually die from cachexia and not the cancer!

Among critically ill postoperative patients, many were found to have magnesium deficiency based on ionized magnesium levels in red blood cells. In one study of patients from a medical intensive care unit (ICU), 65% had low magnesium levels. The author concluded: 'The prevalence of Mg deficiency in critically ill patients may be even higher than 65%, and may lead to hypocalcemia, cardiac arrhythmias and other symptoms of Mg deficiency'.

The following are the key points from an article titled Geriatric cachexia: a role for magnesium deficiency as well as for cytokines?

1. Cachexia's is caused by inflammatory molecules: Prostaglandin E2 and cytokines (IL-1, IL-6, TNF-α) drive inflammation, worsening muscle loss and metabolism.
2. Free radicals amplify the inflammation and damage, while magnesium deficiency further reduces antioxidant defenses.
3. Cytokines choke off appetite. This leads to nausea, vomiting, and disrupted

digestion contribute which causes weight loss alongside muscle breakdown.

4. Anorexia, infections, ulcers, and cognitive decline form a web of devastating complications.

5. Magnesium deficiency fuels the fire of increased inflammatory mediators and free radicals which worsen cachexia in magnesium-deficient individuals.

6. The cytokine substance P, which increases early in magnesium deficiency, may lead to oxidative injury and appetite suppression, possibly contributing to the reduced food intake and weight loss that characteristically occur in experimental animals within 2 weeks of dietary magnesium restriction.

7. Magnesium replacement offers a potential ray of hope. Addressing magnesium deficiency may offer a novel therapeutic approach for cachexia by dampening inflammation and oxidative stress.

Alcohol consumption and cancer both deplete magnesium, and I suspect that the rapid excretion of magnesium while drinking may be the reason excessive alcohol consumption can cause dizziness and black outs and falls. This is a common sever symptom of magnesum deficiency. Possibly supplementing with magnesium while drinking might prevent these side effects.

What are good ways to boost your magnesium levels? Taking a supplement twice a day might be a good start. I have been taking extended-release magnesium 250 mg every day (from www.lef.org) along with 144 mg magnesium threonate in the evening. (Note-You will later see this was too low for me!) You can also purchase bottles of magnesium oil spray for about $10. I spray about 10 squirts on my shoulders and arms every day after I get out of the shower. The oil is something similar to Theramax which is being advertised to stop muscle cramps all over TV. Theramax is primarily a magnesium sulfate spray where if you spray it on your cramped muscle you get relief. For extreme situations there is available a micronized magnesium liquid that you can sip throughout the day to boost your magnesium levels. And finally, even though our foods have less and less magnesium in them, you can still add more of the highest magnesium containing foods to your diet to get your diet pointed in the right direction.

Magnesium Rich Foods:
Almonds, Avocado, Bananas, Black beans, Bran or Shredded Wheat cereal, Brown rice, Cashews, Edamame, Kidney beans, Oatmeal, Peanut butter, Peanuts, Potato with skin, Pumpkin, Raisins, Soymilk, Spinach, Whole grain bread. Also, buying

organic increases the chances that you will be getting a higher magnesium content in your foods

At this point we have probably figured out the cause of and how to prevent about 95% of the modern-day common diseases known to man. This can be done simply by making sure you have plenty of Vitamin D3 and magnesium in your system.

However, there is one more main culprit that leads to a few more diseases, some of them deadly, and is caused by another deficiency in our diet. I am talking about widespread Vitamin K2 deficiency which we will tackle in the next Chapter.

So, you are going to supplement with much higher amounts of magnesium? It would be good to know and look for any of these symptoms of taking too much magnesium: Diarrhea, nausea and vomiting, lethargy, muscle weakness, abnormal electrical conduction in the heart, low blood pressure, urine retention, respiratory distress, cardiac arrest. The good news is the first symptom is diarrhea so if you just increase your dosing in a measured manner, and listen to your body and use diarrhea as an initial warning sign of taking too much magnesium there is almost no chance you will progress to the other symptoms.

Vitamin K2 Deficiency-

I have heard from many people who asked their doctor about Vitamin K2 and in the vast majority of cases the doctor had never heard of it (even a doctor who wrote a thesis paper on Vitamin D3)!

Vitamin D3 is intimately involved with Vitamin K2 as you will see. In the cases where doctors had even heard of Vitamin K2, they usually had no idea what it did. They were usually just vaguely aware that the almost unrelated Vitamin K1 was important for blood clotting.

In the modern era we have unwittingly given almost everyone who lives in the industrialized world, a Vitamin K2 deficiency.

How did this happen? We switched from small farm- pasture raising and grazing of animals, to factory -like mass production farming of animals. Instead of letting them graze on the spring and summer grass as in more agrarian cultures, we put them in pens inside a barn and feed them corn.

So now you will know the secret health benefits of milk from pasture-raised cows, or "grass fed" beef which costs more than regular beef. Why is it healthier? Due to its increased Vitamin K2 content. But you can't just feed any old grass to the animals, a lot of grass does not contain the Vitamin K2 precursors, like fall and winter grass. The grass that does the trick has to be grown during the sunny spring and summer months. (You can pay more for summer grass fed beef and dairy products, or you could just start taking a K2 supplement and eat factory beef and dairy and save some money).

Why is this a problem? Well despite factory farming's cruelty, the animals are no longer getting the precursor to Vitamin K2 found in green grass and plants that grow in the spring and summer. So, this drops the Vitamin K2 content of animal products that we consume to very low levels. This in turn makes us all deficient. Why?

For whatever reason, like our inability to make Vitamin C, humans lost the ability to make enough of our own K2 to allow for good health, and we have to rely on animal and plant sources to get it. Our primary sources of K2 have been from animal products like beef, milk and dairy products, but it can be found in fermented vegetable foods like sauerkraut and Japanese Natto (fermented soybeans-sky high in the MK7 type of K2).

What does Vitamin K2 do? It allows synthesis of and charges up a protein-hormone called osteocalcin that takes the calcium out of your blood and soft tissues and puts it back in your bones. This is critically important when you are boosting your Vitamin D3 levels. Without sufficient K2 levels in your system while you are taking or making higher doses of Vitamin D3- the Vitamin D3 can in some rare cases lead to hypercalcemia. This is caused by Vitamin D3 triggering the accelerated remodeling of your bones and joints which releases large amounts of calcium into your blood. But if you have sufficient K2 in your system, this blood borne calcium is quickly shuttled back into your bones and joints where it belongs by the Vitamin K2-charged hormone osteocalcin.

What is the result of Vitamin K2 deficiency? For starters, due to reduced calcium deposition in the bones, children's jaw bones often don't grow big enough to accommodate all the incoming teeth. Widespread K2 deficiency in childhood has created the orthodontics industry, a needlessly large $12 billion per year business in the US.

A dentist by the name of Weston Price traveled the world to find out why industrialized people had such bad teeth. He found that most indigenous island people had perfect teeth no cavities and almost never needed braces, and they didn't even brush their teeth! They had no idea what floss was and at most engaged in occasional tongue scraping to prevent bad breath. He identified some substance in their food as Factor X. Well it turns out that Factor X was Vitamin K2.

Having proper levels of K2 in one's system will not only prevent your children from needing braces but will prevent them from getting cavities. When you have enough K2 in your system your body will easily deposit calcium where it is needed.

These seem like minor issues compared to the diseases associated with Vitamin D3 deficiency. So, where's the beef?

Vitamin K2 is also essential for preventing some major killers –

Heart disease and atherosclerosis. By keeping calcium from building up in your heart and arteries, Vitamin K2 can prevent this major killer. It works synergistically with magnesium and Vitamin D3.

Aortic Valve Stenosis (Calcification of your major heart valve!) Also, a major killer and heart valve replacement surgery is a big business! All you need to do to avoid this is to boost your K2 levels

Osteoporosis and bone health Vitamin K2 also is very important for bone health and low K2 levels have been found to cause increase the risk of fractures and osteoporosis.

Reduced Cancer Risk

Vitamin K2 has a major role in preventing cancer.

A study published in the March 2010 issue of the American Journal of Clinical Nutrition, found high intake of Vitamin K2—not K1—leads to reduced cancer risk, as well as a **thirty percent lower risk of dying from cancer**

A study funded by the National Cancer Institute found that Vitamin K2 might help reduce the risk for non-Hodgkin lymphoma. Mayo Clinic researchers discovered that people with the highest intake of Vitamin K2 had **a 45 percent lower risk** for this type of cancer, compared to those with the lowest Vitamin K2 intake. Scientists attribute this to the important role that Vitamin K2 plays in inhibiting inflammatory cytokines, which are related to this type of lymphoma, and Vitamin K2's role in the life cycle of your cells.

Prostate cancer   Additionally, an observational study in 11,000 men found that a high Vitamin K2 intake was linked to **a 63% lower risk of advanced prostate cancer**, whereas Vitamin K1 had no effect.

Interestingly, I stumbled upon a little study where they compared men who had some calcification in a certain part of the prostate (peripheral zone) to men who didn't. Of all the men in the study who later developed prostate cancer, they almost all came from the group who had calcification. Vitamin K2 probably works to prevent cancer by preventing calcification of this part of the prostate which seems to be the initiating event for prostate cancer.

179

Here is the title of the study if you are interested:
Prevalence of prostatic calcification subtypes and association with prostate cancer.
Urology. 2015 Jan;85(1):178-81.

Note-Vitamin K2 probably works in concert with Vitamin D3 to prevent prostate cancer as it turns out that the higher Vitamin D3 levels men have, the lower their risk of prostate cancer. Or, it is possible that high levels of Vitamin D3 are actually just a marker for high levels of Vitamin K2. (Studies are needed to clarify this issue please.)

Various items of interest-

- In one study spanning 7–10 years, people with the highest intake of Vitamin K2 were **52% less** likely to develop artery calcification and had a **57% lower** risk of dying from heart disease.
- Another study in 16,057 women found that participants with the highest intake of Vitamin K2 had a much lower risk of heart disease — **for every 10 mcg of K2** they consumed per day, heart disease risk was reduced by 9%
- Vitamin K1 had no influence in either of those studies.
- A 3-year study in 244 postmenopausal women found that those taking Vitamin K2

supplements had much slower decreases in age-related bone mineral density.

- Long-term studies in Japanese women have observed **similar benefits for osteoporosis** - though **very high doses** were used in these cases (45 mg (=45,000 mcg) per day). Out of 13 studies, only one failed to show significant improvement.
- Seven of these trials, which took fractures into consideration, found that Vitamin K2 reduced spinal fractures by **60%,** hip fractures by **77%** and all non-spinal fractures by **81%!** In line with these findings, Vitamin K2 supplements are officially recommended for preventing and treating osteoporosis in Japan.

Finally, it is now becoming known that you can actually reverse arterial calcification by taking high doses of Vitamin K2 (along with D3). Because K2 has no known toxicity, high doses have been used. In Japan they have used 45,000 mcg or 45 milligrams per day for osteoporosis while the typical Vitamin K2 supplement in the US usually contains only 400 mcg of the MK7 type of K2.

I personally have taken 45 mg of K2, 3X per day for 3 months in an effort to decalcify my arteries with no side effects. I also heard from a friend who started taking higher dose vitamin D3 and K2 and after 1 year of this, his doctor told him his latest CT scan showed that his arterial calcifications had completely cleared up.

NOW HERE IS THE MOST IMPORTANT THING YOU CAN LEARN ABOUT VITAMIN K2 IF YOU ARE GOING TO TAKE HIGH DOSE VITAMIN D3-

Doctors have long had an inordinate fear about people taking effective doses of Vitamin D3 ("high") because they have heard of a few (quite rare) cases of Vitamin D toxicity! And this completely clouds their judgment.

I bet you ask- I thought Vitamin D3 was harmless at any dose- so what is Vitamin D toxicity?

Yes-you are right, I did tell you that before, and Vitamin D3 is actually harmless at any dose; D3 is simply information for your genes that is almost always beneficial. However, one thing that Vitamin D3 can do is to accelerate the remodeling process of your bones and joints. This remodeling leads to a release of calcium into your blood, and if everything was working right the calcium would just be deposited back into your bones where it belongs.

But when the calcium is being put back into your bones, your body is eating up the limited amount of functioning Vitamin K2 in your system. Once your K2 is all gone, then the calcium in your blood can increase to dangerous levels and cause what they call "Vitamin D toxicity" also known as hypercalcemia. So, if you decide to take high dose Vitamin D3 you must also supplement with Vitamin K2 just like you have to supplement with magnesium.

The simple solution? Just take as much Vitamin K2 as the high dose Vitamin D3 and your problem is solved. I know a man who has been taking 1 million IUs of D3 per day for over a year for his MS with no problems. His blood calcium remains in the low range. Why? Because he takes a large amount of Vitamin K2 with his D3 which recharges the osteocalcin hormone which is what takes the calcium out of his blood and puts it back in his bones.

In fact, Chris Masterjohn, a Vitamin D and K researcher noticed that most of the symptoms of Vitamin D toxicity were also the same symptoms as Vitamin K2 deficiency. Here is a summary I made of a paper he wrote on the subject:

(While he only identifies it as "Vitamin K" I changed all the Vitamin K references in his abstract to Vitamin K2 for clarification.)

Vitamin D3 toxicity redefined: Vitamin K2 and the molecular mechanism. Med Hypotheses 2007;68(5):1026-34. Masterjohn C.

Major Points of his paper:

- Some recommended Vitamin D3 doses for optimal therapy exceed safety limits.

- Conventional "hypercalcemia" explanation for Vitamin D3 toxicity may be incomplete.

- This hypothesis proposes Vitamin K2 deficiency as a potential alternative mechanism.

- Excessive D3 upregulates proteins needing K2-dependent activation, depleting the K2 pool.

- K2 deficiency symptoms align very closely with observed Vitamin D3 "toxicity" symptoms (anorexia, lethargy, etc.)

- Vitamin K2 deficiency and D3 toxicity share similar features with the effects of Warfarin (a K2 inhibitor).

- Combining D3 with K2 may unlock its full therapeutic potential.

And finally, if you are going to do your own high dose Vitamin K2 experimentation you might want to avoid paying the ridiculous prices that Vitamin K2 pill sellers charge for tiny amounts of K2. Some sellers charge a price that equates to $6500 per gram or about 30 times the price of gold!

You can get pure powder Vitamin K2, both the MK4 (animal/human form) type of K2 and the stronger but less natural MK7 type of K2 from bacterial sources for just $15 per gram! You can go to TakeD3.com and read about Peter at Vitaspace.com's pure powder supplement products. He also is a low cost, highest quality supplier of Vitamin D3, magnesium, and a whole host of anti-aging hormones. You can read a more detailed article about him here at this link>>>

https://jefftbowles.com/how-to-save-90percent-and-more-on-vitamins-hormones-supplements/

One last note-I had seen comments by a number of people who were taking just Vitamin K2, and some said it made their heart race, especially if they were taking the stronger MK-7 type of K2. This sounds like K2 was also inducing a magnesium deficiency. Possibly K2 allows the body to put more magnesium into one's bones thus triggering the heart symptoms. An alternate explanation might be that it transfers so much calcium from the blood to the bone that heart rhythm disturbances could be triggered.

Good News: So far, Vitamin K2 has no known toxicity at any dose.

Boron Deficiency-

I originally was going to publish this book describing the 3 deadly deficiencies of the modern age- Vitamin D3, magnesium, and Vitamin K2. But then I started thinking about the fact that high doses of Vitamin D3 seemed to eat up large amounts of magnesium and Vitamin K2, and if they were not replaced, then high dose Vitamin D3 could become harmful due to causing or exacerbating K2 or magnesium deficiencies.

So, I asked myself, is there anything else that high dose Vitamin D3 might cause our bodies to consume at a higher rate than normal? The answer was simple- just look at the list of major cofactors for Vitamin D3. They include:

Magnesium.... check
Vitamin K2.... check
Boron
Zinc
Vitamin A (do not take the retinol form of Vitamin A with D3 but instead take beta carotene- more on this later).

I started looking at boron expecting to find lots of research on this Vitamin D3 cofactor. I was surprised; almost all the research done on boron concerns plant diseases caused by boron deficient soil. I could initially find no estimates as to how many people were boron deficient.

186

What I did find was the interesting work of a man named Rex E. Newnham who was an English plant scientist who studied boron deficiency in plants. He found that after he moved to Australia to continue his research, he all of the sudden developed arthritis. Knowing that the area where he lived had boron deficient soil, he experimented on himself by taking 30 mg of boron two times a day in the form of Borax laundry powder which was sold as a cleaning agent to whiten your laundry. Borax powder simply consisted of 4 molecules of boron attached to a sodium molecule. He was very excited to find his arthritis cleared up in a few months. He then embarked on making tablets from Borax and selling them to others in Australia with arthritis. Within 5 years, and solely by word of mouth, he was selling 10,000 bottles a month! He made the mistake of approaching a drug company to see if they were interested, and after they realized they could not patent the supplement they reported him to the government. The government quickly outlawed the sale of Borax in Australia! That was pretty much the end of Rex's story except for a few research articles he published.

He did some research and basically discovered that in countries or areas with boron poor soil, that the rates of arthritis were as high as 70% where even the dogs got arthritis. While in areas with high levels of boron in the soil arthritis rates were 0 to 10% of the population.

He also heard some stories from doctors who noticed that when they had to cut the bones of regular patients it was relatively easy, but cutting the bones of people who supplemented with boron was much more difficult due to their bones' amazing hardness and strength. He also noted the case of an 87-year-old woman who was a regular boron user who fell down a long flight of stairs. To everyone's amazement she didn't have a single broken bone after the fall.

Here is a summary of two papers he wrote for some science journals:

Agricultural practices affect arthritis.
Nutr Health. 1991;7(2):89-100. Newnham RE.
Summary:
- Boron deficiency in food might be linked to arthritis prevalence.
- Studies suggest soil depletion by fertilizers impacts boron levels in crops.
- Countries with low boron intake (e.g., maize-based diets) show higher arthritis rates.
- Boron levels in food have dwindled globally, potentially contributing to rising arthritis cases, including juvenile cases.
- Fertilizer and plant selection practices may be altering nutrient content in food, with

boron deficiency potentially signaling broader nutritional losses.

Essentiality of boron for healthy bones and joints.
Environ Health Perspect.1994 Nov;102 Suppl 7:83-5.Newnham RE –

- Growing evidence suggests boron can safely and effectively treat certain forms of arthritis.
- Personal experience spurred investigation, followed by diverse research:
    - Lower boron levels found in bones and joint fluids of arthritis patients.
    - Supplemented bones observed to be sturdier.
    - Epidemiological studies: Countries with high boron intake have lower arthritis rates.
    - Animal and human trials: Boron showed positive effects on arthritic symptoms.
- These findings suggest boron is an essential nutrient for bone and joint health.
- Further research is warranted to explore boron's potential in treating and preventing arthritis.

Boron and Arthritis: The Results of a Double-blind Pilot Study. Journal of Nutritional & Environmental Medicine 1(2):127-132 · July 2009 Newham et. al.

Boron for Osteoarthritis: A Promising Pilot Study

A small, double-blind study suggests boron may be effective in treating osteoarthritis.

- Trial: 20 patients received either 6mg daily boron or placebo.
- Results: 71% of those who completed the trial on boron improved (50% of those who started the trial on boron improved)
- Placebo: Only 10% of those starting the trial on placebo improved.
- Side effects: None reported.
- Conclusion: Boron appears safe and beneficial for osteoarthritis; further research needed.

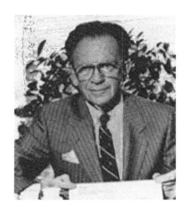

Rex Newnham

Rex Newnham passed away in 2010 at age 90. Sadly, his work just seems to have stopped and not been picked up by anyone. In the meantime, as is their general modus operandi, various governments around the world have banished Borax from being sold to the public.

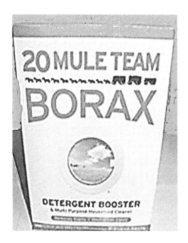

Countries that have banned the sale of Borax include the European union, Australia, China, and Thailand to name a few. Instead, 3 mg boron supplements are now available for people who want to supplement with boron, quite a smaller dose than the 60 mg a day that Newnham was taking. Remember however that borax is only 11% boron by weight so the 60 mg dose Newnham was taking was equivalent to 6.6 mg of elemental boron.

Also keep in mind that borax is reported to be less toxic than table salt.

What are the health risks associated with boron deficiency?

-ankylosing spondylitis
-arthritis
-bone density- low
-bone development- abnormal
-calcium excretion- increased urinary
-embryonic development problems
-growth- impaired
-immune function- low
-osteoporosis- high incidence of
-rheumatoid arthritis
-tooth decay
-wound healing- impaired

Other interesting facts about boron:

- Boron **increases the useful life of Vitamin D3** in your system.
- Boron **helps your body absorb magnesium**.
- In areas of Australia where water and soil levels of boron are high, half the cases of musculoskeletal diseases have been reported when compared with areas containing lower boron levels.
- Country by country comparisons found that arthritis rates decrease as boron levels in the

soil increase. Which leads to an increase of boron in the food supply.

- One study found that 3 percent boric acid applied to deep wounds **reduced healing time by almost 70%!** This is because boron activates skin and tissue wound healing cells called fibroblasts in a manner similar to its action on osteoblasts.
- The body needs boron to create and maintain a good balance the sex hormones estrogen and testosterone, boron increases both T and E levels.
- Most boron deficiency symptoms overlap with D3 deficiency symptoms.
- Boron keeps your teeth and gums healthy by stimulating bone and tissue repair and reducing inflammation.
- A boron paste accelerated healing of foot ulcers in diabetics.
- Boron deficiency can lead to osteoporosis and rickets.
- Boron enhances major mineral content in bone, and, independently of vitamin D3, enhances cartilage remodeling which implies that D3 and boron both belong to a larger multi-factor metabolic system.
- Boron deficiency causes impaired bone healing because of reduced osteogenesis (bone cell formation).

- Arthritic bones contain less boron than healthy bones
- Boron reduces the cytokines which are involved with causing lung and breast cancers, insulin resistance, coronary disease, depression and obesity.
- Some boron compounds, such as borax and boric acid, prevented DNA damage from dangerous heavy metals like lead, arsenic, and mercury in cell studies.
- Boron may be especially helpful in preventing prostate cancer by suppressing the levels of PSA in the prostate.
- Brain activity such as attention span and short-term memory, as well as coordination are decreased in boron deficient animals and people.
- Boron with Vitamin B6 and water can help eliminate kidney stones, 10mg/day increased kidney stone elimination and decreased pain from passing the stones.
- Boron supplements also increased the mineral density of athletes' bones.
- Boron prevents DNA damage and in turn cancer initiation.

Dr. Newnham also observed improvements in arthritic dogs treated with boric acid.

Because there has been little to no research on the dietary needs for boron the USDA and other "authorities" have come up with an "upper limit" where they know no one has had any negative effects from too much boron. They have not even bothered to come up with a minimum recommended daily allowance

Based on what we know about the ridiculous daily recommended intake of Vitamin D3, these boron recommendations could be way too low. Boron is less toxic than table salt. Let us compare the USDA's recommendations for boron vs. table salt.

BORON-upper limits

1-3 years old	3 mg
4-8 Years	6 mg
9-13 years	11 mg
14-18 years	17 mg
Adults 19-50 years	20 mg
Pregnant women	17-20 mg
Women who are Breast feeding	20-25 mg

SALT- adequate vs upper limits

	adequate	upper
0-6 months	120 mg	no data
7-12 months	370 mg	no data
1-3 years old	1,000 mg	1,500 mg
4-8 Years	1,200 mg	1,900 mg

9-13 years	1,500 mg	2,200 mg
Adults 14-50 years	1,500 mg	2,300 mg
Older Adults 51-70yrs	1,300 mg	2,300 mg
Older Adults over 70	1,200 mg	2,300 mg

Regarding the above guidelines, for some reason they focus on age as a proxy for weight! Why not just make the limits based on weight! How stupid!

Also, do you think the snack manufacturers had anything to do with the salt numbers!!??

So, isn't that interesting? The daily recommended allowance for boron intake is 1/75th of that of table salt. This, while the toxic dose of table salt is 25 grams, and the toxic dose for boron is 50 grams!

I think the daily healthy dose for boron needs to be looked into. This could be another scandal waiting to be uncovered just like the Vitamin D3 intake guideline scandal.

The boron content of the world's farmland has likely been declining since the beginning of farming. Of modern societies, France has the highest average daily boron intake of 10/mg per day while the average intake in the UK is .8 to 5.0 mg/day. As expected, France has half the rate of rheumatoid arthritis and ankylosing spondylitis as in the UK.

US average intake is 1.5 mg per day, and in Canada only 1.2 mg per day!

In boron-rich regions of Turkey drinking water sources with 29 mg boron/liter are consumed without harmful effects.

I feel quite comfortable taking 30 mg of boron 2X a day and will continue to do so.

My anecdotal report about my experience with higher dose boron for both me and my dog follows:

My 13-year old German Shepherd, Sasha, and I have only been taking higher dose boron for about six weeks now. What I CAN TELL YOU IS THAT IN THE FIRST TWO WEEKS I SAW A PROFOUND DIFFERENCE IN MY OLD GERMAN SHEPHERD who is already about a year older than almost all German Shepherds live. (I have been giving her every anti-aging supplements I know for the last 4 or 5 years).

The major change I noticed in her was that her arthritic back hips and legs really seemed to loosen up quite a bit after just a few days of boron supplementation.

Before the boron, she would normally just want to sleep most of the day, and only go out once a day on the porch to do her business But after a few days of 30 mg of Boron 2X per day   she was going out down the stairs to go outside for a short walk every day. And she had earlier gotten to the point where she almost never wanted to get into my truck to go for a ride anymore. She had always wanted to go trucking when she was younger.

In the first week of boron supplementation she got into the truck 5 out of 7 days! This has tapered off a bit, but she still likes to go for a ride about 3X per week. Also, before I put her on the boron regimen she almost never wanted to go up and down the stairs from the first floor to the second floor anymore. She would just sleep on the first floor every night. Since being on boron, she comes upstairs to sleep every night, and some days goes up and down the stairs as many as 5 times! Also, the boron seemed to have some sort of mental effects on her as well, as she stated playing with her tennis ball again after about a year of ignoring it.

As far as I go after the first four years or so after my high dose Vitamin D3 experiment, both of my shoulders were healed from old injuries and were in perfect shape, but after the four years of grace, I acquired what seemed like a frozen right shoulder. I somehow thought it was connected with the high dose D3, that maybe it was some sort of evolved long-term healing process meant to immobilize your arm like a sling while the shoulder was being remodeled. But it has lasted for several years and I still have it to this day. This has prevented me from lifting anywhere near heavy weights for exercise; I have been barely even able to do a push up due to pain for some time. Within just a few days of taking higher dose boron I noticed a definite big improvement in my shoulder. I have started lifting light weights again. I was hoping for a continuation of the miracle after the first week or two, but it quickly plateaued and my progress after the first two weeks was much slower. So that is where I am after about 6 weeks, at a plateau, waiting for longer term progress which I hope will continue. I will post updates to this boron experiment to my website jeffTbowles.com from time to time if you want to check back.

Wait! I now have an amazing update! I have been taking high dose boron for about 7 weeks now, but the last week I started taking a lot more magnesium than before and high dose zinc. Before I had assumed that I was taking enough magnesium, 250 mg per day of extended release magnesium from lef.org. I have also been spraying about 10 to 12 sprays of magnesium oil on my skin after my shower. I have also been taking 144 mg of magnesium threonate at night. I also have had a diet high in magnesium rich foods like almonds, peanuts, other nuts, and hummus etc. Also, I had done a month-long magnesium replenishment routine as promoted by Dr. Carolyn Dean that included micro magnesium liquid about a year ago. I thought I have been taking enough!

But now I realize I was still magnesium deficient!

I feel like a total idiot! Why? Because I have been experimenting for about 4 years to try and fix my frozen shoulder/tendonitis, and have gotten no dramatic results, which has prevented me from lifting weights which has been part of my routine since high school!

So just yesterday, October 16, 2019, after supplementing with boron for 6 weeks, then adding high dose zinc and increasing my magnesium intake by about 500% per a week, a massage therapist was able to push my arm up over my head until I heard first one muffled pop, then another, and then two more. A total of four adhesions were broken. (Frozen shoulder is also known as adhesive capsulitis). After each pop my arm was able to move further and further! After we were done, my range of motion increased from about 70% to maybe 90%! Apparently, we ripped away calcium adhesions between my tendon and my bone and freed up the shoulder! Now my shoulder feels much looser but the day after the "pops", it feels like the shoulder has been slightly sprained, no longer sharp pains, but more of a dull ache, with lots more mobility!

I then searched BING for magnesium and frozen shoulder and what did I find? A website called the tendonitis expert who is adamant that frozen shoulder and or tendonitis is caused by magnesium deficiency! And he has 10 years+ of experience, lots of satisfied clients, has written many books on the subject, and makes fun of doctors who don't know how to cure it-my kind of guy!

Why do I feel so stupid? Because I have been advising people at least every week that if they have any bad reactions after taking high dose Vitamin D3 that there is about a 99% chance that it is caused by aggravating an underlying magnesium deficiency! For some reason I thought it only applied to short-term negative effects, **but now I realize high dose Vitamin D3 induced magnesium deficiency can strike at any time! Even years after starting the D3 regimen** as we saw with the nuclear scientist in the Vitamin D3-bad reactions chapter. How did I not see this!!?? Four years of weightlifting down the drain! However, in all fairness, I was never sure that it was frozen shoulder, as it occurred where I had had old injuries when younger and nowhere else.

Was it the boron, or the addition of high dose magnesium, the zinc or a combination of the three?

I don't know. According to the tendonitis expert, website- www.TendonitisExpert.com , he claims that magnesium directs your body to absorb errant calcium deposits. It has generally been presumed that this was the job of Vitamin K2, apparently magnesium performs this function as well, maybe a little differently.

The Bing search for magnesium and frozen shoulder also displays a page called:

5 Powerful Natural Remedies for Frozen Shoulder. The first remedy is listed as **magnesium and boron.** The second remedy is listed as **Vitamin D3 and K2**.

Also having my 4-year frozen shoulder loosen up exactly on the same day I finish this book! What are the odds of that??!

Symptoms of Excessive Boron Intake Include:

Skin inflammation and peeling, irritability, tremors, convulsions, weakness, headaches, depression, diarrhea, vomiting- I don't have any of these yet!

Zinc Deficiency-

Like magnesium. boron, and Vitamin K2, zinc is an important cofactor of Vitamin D3. Just as high dose Vitamin D3 depletes Vitamin K2 and magnesium stores, I believe it is quite likely that it also depletes our bodies of boron and zinc as well. All these cofactors are enlisted by Vitamin D3 to increase thousands of metabolic and enzymatic reactions in the body.

Just like magnesium and boron, it is estimated that about half the world's farmland is deficient in zinc. This leads to the current situation where up to **1/3 of the world's population is zinc deficient**. Severe zinc deficiency is rare, but mild and moderate zinc deficiencies are quite common. It is also estimated that **in the US** 12% of the general population is zinc deficient and **40% are zinc deficient** if you look at just the elderly demographic. Most of the deficiencies are caused by growing crops in zinc deficient soil. Zinc fertilization not only increases zinc content in zinc deficient crops, it also increases crop yields. There ought to be a law!

The recommended daily allowance for zinc is about 10 mg per day for adults, but keep in mind these minimum recommended amounts are usually just enough to keep you from getting obvious diseases. The tolerable upper **intake** level (UL) for **zinc** at **40**

mg per day for adults has been set by health "authorities".

The food highest in zinc is by far oysters followed by beans and nuts. Exercising, high alcohol intake, and diarrhea all increase loss of zinc from the body.

Zinc deficiency is thought to be the leading cause of infant mortality Because the thymus needs a lot of zinc to function properly, children with zinc-starved thymuses will have malfunctioning immune systems and be much more likely to die of dysfunction of the immune system, chronic diarrhea and/or acute respiratory infections

Over 300 zinc containing enzymes have been identified, as well as over 1000 zinc containing transcription factors.

Now here is the cool stuff:

Zinc is the fourth cofactor that helps Vitamin D3 do its work. I have always known there is something special about zinc, as in my early years of studying aging one of the first amazing facts I learned was that as all vertebrate animals age, their thymus glands shrink to a very small size even at a young age. It is called thymic involution. At one year of age the human thymus starts shrinking about 3% per year until we reach the age of about 40, and then the shrinkage drops to about 1% a year.

The thymus is a gland in your neck that is an important part of your immune system that makes T-cells some of which kill virus infected cells and cancer cells. Other T-cells are called suppressor cells because they prevent the immune system from attacking the "self" or good tissues. Vitamin D3 both revs up your killer immune system and suppresses any attacks on the good tissues of the self. So, you can bet that the thymus and Vitamin D3 are very much intimately linked. The thymus is supposed to work until age 105 theoretically but it was shown however that most people over 40 cannot create brand new T cells (naïve) in response to encountering never seen before viruses. It was also shown that in the elderly, thymus size was inversely correlated with cancer rates, autoimmune diseases and infections.

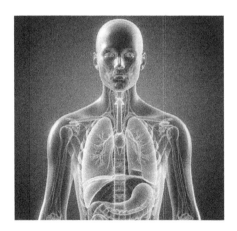

The amazing thing about zinc that I learned was that when they give both zinc and melatonin to mice, their thymuses regrew!

From J Neuroimmunol. 1994 Sep;53(2):189-201. The immuno-reconstituting effect of melatonin or pineal grafting and its relation to zinc pool in aging mice. (my note the pineal graft is melatonin-producing tissue) It has been demonstrated that melatonin, the main neuro-hormone of the pineal gland, affects thymic functions and the regulation of the immune system. In addition, experimental evidences indicate that **melatonin can modulate zinc turnover**. The knowledge that **with advancing age both melatonin and zinc plasma levels decline**, and that **zinc supplementation in old mice is able to restore the reduced immunological functions**, has prompted investigations on the effect of chronic melatonin treatment or pineal graft in old mice on the age-related decline of thymic endocrine activity, peripheral immune functions and zinc turnover. Both **melatonin treatment** in old mice and pineal graft **into the thymus of old mice correct the reduced thymic endocrine activity and increase the weight of the thymus** and its cellularity. A restoration of cortical thymic volume, as detected by the percentage of tissue in active proliferation, is also observed in old mice after both treatments.

Thymocyte CD phenotype expression is also restored to young values. At peripheral level, recovery of peripheral blood lymphocyte number and of spleen cell subsets, with increased mitogen responsiveness also occurs. **Melatonin treatment or pineal graft induce also a restoration of the altered zinc turnover in aged mice with an increment of the crude zinc balance from negative (-1.6 microgram/day/mouse) to positive value (+1.2 microgram/day/mouse), similar to that one of young mice** (+1.4 microgram/ day/ mouse). The reduced zinc plasma level is restored to normal values. These findings support the idea that the effect of melatonin on thymic endocrine activity and peripheral immune functions may be mediated by the zinc pool.

And from Plasticity of neuroendocrine-thymus interactions during aging-

Thymic regrowth and reactivation of thymic endocrine activity may be achieved even in old animals by different endocrinological or nutritional manipulations such as, (a) intrathymic transplantation of pineal gland **or treatment with melatonin**, (b) implantation of a growth hormone (GH) secreting tumor cell line or treatment with exogenous GH, (c) castration or treatment with exogenous luteinizing hormone-releasing hormone (LH-RH), (d) treatment with exogenous thyroxine or triiodothyronine, and (e**) nutritional interventions such as arginine or zinc**

supplementation. These data strongly suggest that thymic involution is a phenomenon secondary to age-related alterations in neuroendocrine-thymus interactions and that it is the disruption of such interactions in old age that is responsible for age-associated dysfunction. **Melatonin** or other pineal factors may act through specific receptors, but experimental evidence is still lacking. **The role of zinc, whose turnover is usually reduced in old age, is diverse. The effects range from the reactivation of zinc-dependent enzymes, required for both cell proliferation and apoptosis, to the reactivation of thymulin, a zinc-dependent thymic hormone. The role of zinc may even be more crucial.** According to recent preliminary data obtained both in animal and human studies, it appears that the above reported **endocrinological manipulations capable of restoring thymic activity in old age, may act also by normalizing the altered zinc pool.**

This is great! Apparently at old ages animals like us can regrow our thymuses with zinc and melatonin supplementation and keep our immune systems young!

Melatonin is an amazing anti-aging hormone and if you want to learn more about it you can start with my articles>>

Amazing! Melatonin Secrets That Almost Nobody Knows About! Link>

https://jefftbowles.com/melatonin-secrets-that-almost-nobody-knows-about-amazing/

The 6 Changes in Lifetime Hormone Levels that Cause Aging – And How to Easily Reverse Them! Link>

https://jefftbowles.com/the-6-changes-in-lifetime-hormone-levels-that-cause-aging-and-how-to-easily-reverse-them/

Another amazing fact about zinc that I learned in the past was that if you suck on zinc gluconate lozenges at the first sign of a cold, the length of the cold was supposedly reduced by almost 50%. Sounds very similar to the action of Vitamin D3 no?

So, let's take a look at the zinc deficiency diseases and see if we can notice any patterns? Next to each symptom I have indicated what other deficiencies share the same symptom.

Zinc Deficiency Symptoms and Diseases
& Other Deficiencies Causing Similar Symptoms

Acne	**D3 z**
ADHD	D3 m z
Alopecia (thin and	D3 z

sparse hair)	
Zinc Deficiency Symptoms and Diseases & Other Deficiencies Causing Similar Symptoms	
Anemia	D3 z
Angular cheilitis-sores/corners of mouth	z
Anorexia Nervosa	m z
Appetite-loss of	m z
Appetite poor	m z
Attention- less in neonatal period	D3 m z
Birth- hemorrhage during	z
Birth- labor difficult and prolonged	D3 z
Birthpregncs1abort 2defects	b D3 z
Blood elevated ammonia levels	z
Bowel diseases small int.	D3 z
Depression	D3 z
Diarrhea	m z
Eczema	D3 z
Emotional disturbance	D3 m z
Fatal when extreme	z
Genitalia infantile	z

(zinc reversed)	
Zinc Deficiency Symptoms and Diseases & Other Deficiencies Causing Similar Symptoms	
Growth- delayed in children	b z
Growth- stunted 1/3rd world	b z
Happiness reduced level of	D3 z
Hypogonadism Zinc required4 Test.	D3 z
Infant mortality	D3 z
Infections	D3 z
Infections other	D3 z
Infections Gastrointestinal	D3 z
Infections Respiratory	D3 z
Immune function low	**b D3 m z**
Inflammation chronic	D3 z
Irritability	m z
Kidney disease- chronic	D3 z
Learning Impaired	D3 m z
Fatigue extreme	D3 m z
Liver disease- chronic	z
Photo night blindness	m z
Pneumonia	z
Puberty delayed	b D3 z

Zinc Deficiency Symptoms and Diseases & Other Deficiencies Causing Similar Symptoms	
Schizophrenia-decr. brain zinc levels	D3 z
Sickle cell disease	D3 z
Smell: Reduced sense	z
Stomatitis-canker sore	z
Taste acuity impaired	z
Osteoporosis	**b D3 m z**
Ulceration oral	z
Weight loss extreme	m z
Wilson's disease	z
Wound healing-delayed	b D3 z
Wound healing-impaired	b D3 z
Xerosis (dry scaling skin)	D3 z
Cancer head/neck esophagus	D3 K2 z

The pattern that emerges by comparing **zinc to D3, boron, and magnesium** deficiencies is that a few **symptoms are common to all of the cofactors**: **Osteoporosis** (occurs with K2 deficiency as well) and **Impaired immune function**

212

If you take out boron and see what **D3, mg, and zinc** deficiency symptoms have in common we are left with

Fatigue and
Mental issues

If you take out the magnesium and see what **boron D3 and zinc** have in common you get

Wound healing-delayed,
Growth-delayed,
Puberty-delayed, and
Embryonic development-impaired

Symptoms in common with **D3, K2, and z** deficiencies include
Osteoporosis and various **cancers**.

Symptoms unique to **just D3 and Z** are
Skin and hair diseases,
Infections.

The bottom line here is that you can see that each of these cofactors has a huge interaction with most of the other cofactors, so when you supplement with D3 it is surely wise to add magnesium K2 boron and zinc to the regimen to ensure that you optimize your health.

The following table summarizes most of the foods with significant quantities of zinc, listed in order of quantity per serving, unfortified. Note that all of the top 10 entries are meat, beans, or nuts.

It is interesting to note that oysters are extremely high in zinc and are also alleged to be an aphrodisiac It was rumored that Casanova, the French lothario, ate 50 oysters a day which supposedly helped him service all his ladies. It does seem to make sense due to the fact that zinc is required to produce testosterone, and oysters are by far the food with the highest zinc content.

(this list of foods with the highest levels of zinc is omitted in paperback-please see eBook or email me for the pdf at BannedCovidBook@gmail.com)

Vitamin A- the Bad Apple of the Vitamin D3 Cofactors?

I do **not** recommend supplementing with Vitamin A, especially the pure retinol form of Vitamin A. Taking beta carotene in lieu of retinol is preferable because the body converts beta carotene into Vitamin A on an as needed basis.

What's wrong with Vitamin A you ask?

The main thing is that at even small doses of as little as 3000 IU's a day, it completely negates Vitamin D3's cancer prevention effects!

From Dr. Mercola's excellent website:

"The British Medical Journal has published a remarkable paper confirming that low **Vitamin D3** levels obtained in the past are a risk factor for developing colon cancer in the future.

But the study contained an even more significant finding -- as Dr. Cannell's site has reported before, Vitamin A, even in relatively low amounts, can **counteract** Vitamin D3's association with reduced rates of colon cancer.

This is the largest study to date showing Vitamin A blocks Vitamin D3's effect.

Hidden on page eight of the paper was one sentence and a small table, showing that the **benefits of**

Vitamin D3 are almost entirely negated in those with the highest Vitamin A (retinol) intake.

And the retinol intake did not have to be that high -- only about 3,000 IU/day. Young autistic children often take 3,500 IU of retinol a day in their powdered multivitamins, and this would be in addition to any additional Vitamin A given to them in separate higher dose pills.

The finding explains some of the anomalies in other papers on Vitamin D3 and cancer -- similar studies sometimes have widely different results. This may be because the effect of Vitamin A was not considered. In some countries, cod liver oil, which contains Vitamin A, is commonly used as a Vitamin D3 supplement, and in others it is used more rarely, causing differences in the results.

If you already subscribe to the excellent newsletter from **The Vitamin D Council** then you're aware of this important information. If not, I highly recommend becoming a subscriber, as The Vitamin D Council is a great source of information on this vital topic.

In this recent article by Dr. Cannell, he discusses the **latest research published in the British Medical Journal**, which confirms his previous assertion: that **too much Vitamin A negates many of the beneficial health effects of Vitamin D3**.

In his **December 2008 issue**, Dr. Cannell explained: *"The crux of the problem is that a form of Vitamin A, **retinoic acid**, weakly activates the Vitamin D3 response element on the gene and perhaps blocks Vitamin D3's more robust activation. In fact, the authors of a **1993 study** state "there is a profound inhibition of Vitamin D3-activated...gene expression by retinoic acid."*

So, what does this mean?

Vitamin A versus Vitamin D3

Well, naturally, since appropriate Vitamin D3 levels are crucial for your health, it means that it's essential to have *the proper ratio* of Vitamin D3 to Vitamin A in your body. This also means that **Vitamin A supplementation is potentially hazardous to your overall health**, as Vitamin D3 plays a significant role in a large number of common diseases and afflictions.

There are only 30,000 genes in your body and Vitamin D3 has been shown to influence over 2,000 of them. That's one of the primary reasons it influences so many diseases.

Vitamin A production is tightly controlled in your body. The substrate, or source of the Vitamin A, are carotenoids from vegetables in your intestine. Your body converts these carotenoid substrates to exactly the right amount of retinol. However, **when you**

217

take Vitamin A as retinol directly, such as in cod liver oil, you bypass all the natural controls in this closed system. Even Low Amounts of Vitamin A (retinol) Can Negate Benefits of Vitamin D3.

Ideally, you'll want to provide all the Vitamin A and Vitamin D3 substrate your body needs in such a way that your body can regulate both systems naturally.

This is best done by eating colorful vegetables (for Vitamin A) and by exposing your skin to sun every day (for Vitamin D3). (My note-I agree that some sun is good, but to get to the levels of D3 in your system to bullet proof your health while keeping your skin relatively young looking, I believe everyone will have to take supplements).

Given that cancer, heart disease and diabetes are three of the top causes of death in the United States, ensuring that you are getting enough of this crucial Vitamin (D3) should be a top priority.

A study by Dr. William Grant, Ph.D., another internationally recognized research scientist and Vitamin D3 expert, found that about **30 percent of cancer deaths** -- which amounts to 2 million worldwide and 200,000 in the United States -- could be prevented each year with higher levels of Vitamin D3.

Knowing this, it's clearly important **to avoid anything that might hamper your Vitamin D3 production,** and it appears Vitamin A supplementation may indeed have this effect.

I highly recommend you **read Dr. Cannell's article** about this latest BMJ study, in its entirety, as he explains quite well how even the researchers themselves seem to have missed this crucial connection.

The Synergistic Effects of Vitamin A on Vitamin D

"It's highly unfortunate, but many people in developed countries are potentially sabotaging the multitude of health benefits they could receive from adequate Vitamin D3 by taking excessive amounts of Vitamin A, either in the form of multi-vitamins or cod liver oil.

I spent many hours reviewing this issue in the latter part of 2008, and as a result, I issued a **revision of my long held recommendation for cod liver oil**. If you missed that important update, please take the time to review it now.

I had recommended cod liver oil as a source of Vitamin D3 for quite some time, prior to this revision. My stance was based on the fact that cod liver oil contains vitamins D3 and A in addition to healthy omega-3 fats. These vitamins are essential for most everyone who cannot get regular sun exposure year-round.

However, as I began reviewing the latest research, I realized there was compelling evidence that the *ratios* of these two vitamins may be of paramount importance in order to extract optimal health benefits. And this latest study appears to confirm that theory.

It's important to understand that **Vitamin A is essential for your immune system and a precursor to active hormones** that regulate the expression of your genes just like Vitamin D3, and the two *work in tandem.*

For example, **there is evidence that without Vitamin D3, Vitamin A can be ineffective or even toxic**. But if you're deficient in Vitamin A, Vitamin D3 cannot function properly either.

So proper balance of these two vitamins is essential. Too much or too little of either may create negative consequences.

Unfortunately, we do not yet know the optimal ratios between these two vitamins, but it is clear that nearly all cod liver oil products supply them in levels that do not appear to be ideal. You also need to discern between various forms of Vitamin A.

It is the *retinoic acid (retinol)* form of Vitamin A that is problematic. Not beta carotene. Beta carotene is not a concern because it is PRE-Vitamin A. Your body will simply not over-convert beta carotene to excessive levels of Vitamin A. So, taking beta carotene supplements is not going to interfere with your Vitamin D3. "

Vitamin A deficiency symptoms:
(and other cofactors w/same deficiency symptoms)

Acne Breakouts.	a D3
Dry Eyes.	a
Dry Skin.	a D3
Eye problems	a D3
Growth delayed.	a b D3
Infections- Chest	a D3
Infections- throat	a D3
Infertility	a D3
Night Blindness.	a m
Wound Healing-Impaired	a b D3

Because you only need a small amount of Vitamin A each day you could probably get by with simply eating a carrot or taking a beta carotene supplement to prevent the problems listed above. Or if you take a multi-vitamin make sure it only has beta carotene and no retinol.

While beta carotene does sound like a safe alternative to retinol, you should consider that **the use of beta-carotene has been associated with an <u>increased risk of lung cancer</u>** in people who smoke or who have been exposed to asbestos. One study of 29,000 male smokers found an 18% increase in lung cancer in the group receiving 20 mg of beta-carotene a day for 5 to 8 years. Possibly the Vitamin A produced by the carotene was interfering with Vitamin D3's anti-cancer effects.

So truly be careful when taking Vitamin A.

Symptoms of a single overdose of Vitamin A (retinol) include:

abdominal pain
drowsiness
increased pressure on the brain
irritability
nausea
vomiting
Symptoms of chronic Vitamin A overdosing:
(Oddly these symptoms match many of the symptoms of deficiencies in Vitamin D3 and its other cofactors. This is an area ripe for research-does high dose Vitamin A induce deficiencies in other essential minerals and hormones?)
blurry vision or other vision changes
bone pain

confusion
cracked fingernails
dizziness
dry, rough skin
hair loss
itchy or peeling skin
mouth ulcers
nausea and vomiting
poor appetite
respiratory infection
sensitivity to sunlight
skin cracks at the corners of your mouth (seen in zinc deficiency)
swelling of the bones
yellowed skin (jaundice)
In infants and children, symptoms may also include:
bulging eyeballs
bulging of the soft spot on the top of an infant's skull (fontanel)
coma
double vision
inability to gain weight
softening of the skull bone

The pro-cancer effects of retinol provide a nice segway into to the next chapter-Can High Dose Vitamin D3 cure cancer?

Can High Dose Vitamin D3 Cure Cancer?

From the 1,000+ case reports I have heard about concerning high dose Vitamin D3 supplementation, it is quite clear that high dose Vitamin D3 can cure a long list of autoimmune and other diseases by revving up the immune system to attack bad actors, and to tamp it down in the area of attacking healthy tissues.

Logically, one would expect high dose Vitamin D3 would train the immune system to kill off any cancer cells it encounters as long as they have not picked up too many immortalization mutations. In fact, that is exactly what the new "biologic "drugs are doing in many cases, just revving up one aspect of our immune system to have it identify and attack cancers cells. So, if Vitamin D3 is the ultimate biologic as I proposed, shouldn't it be able to do the job better than any biologic?

I have always predicted that high dose D3 could be used to kill all kinds of cancer cells, even those with many of the immortalization mutations. And while the evidence all points in this direction the case study evidence has been sorely lacking. I believe this might be because most people who get cancer, which is considered much more deadly than autoimmune diseases, are in such a panic that they don't think about trying D3. They feel better putting their lives in the hands of the "smart" doctors with their chemotherapy, surgery, and radiation treatments to poison, cut out' or fry the deadly cancer cells. I believe most people do not try high dose D3 for cancer because they basically go into full panic mode.

Let's look at some amazing facts about Vitamin D3 and cancer and then see if we can't find any case studies out there.

Here are some amazing study conclusions:

Every 10 nanograms per milliliter (ng/ml) increase in blood D3 levels could translate to a 29% reduction in cancer death rates. This means a simple adjustment in your D3 intake could have a significant impact on overall cancer risk.

Colorectal cancer stands out as particularly susceptible to D3's influence. Studies suggest that higher D3 levels may lead to a 49% decrease in death rates from this prevalent form of cancer.

Seasonality plays a role, too. A Norwegian study revealed that cancer patients diagnosed in summer, when D3 levels peak, enjoyed 40% better survival rates compared to those diagnosed in winter when D3 levels plummet. This highlights the potential benefit of optimizing D3 levels throughout the year.

For breast cancer patients, the fight becomes personal. Low D3 levels were linked to a 70%

increased risk of death over 11 years, alongside double the rate of metastasis compared to those with adequate D3 levels. This underscores the importance of D3 screening and potential supplementation for breast cancer patients.

Even in lung cancer, the D3 effect shines through. Early-stage patients diagnosed in summer with high D3 levels had a five-year survival rate of 73%, compared to a mere 30% for those diagnosed in winter with low D3 levels. These findings suggest that maintaining optimal D3 levels could significantly improve lung cancer outcomes.

The benefits extend beyond specific cancers. High D3 levels are linked to a reduced risk of developing various malignancies, including lung, colon, prostate, renal, and endometrial cancers. It seems D3 casts a broad protective net over our health.

Even in advanced stages of colorectal cancer, D3 offers hope. High D3 levels were found to reduce the risk of death by over 60% compared to patients with low D3 levels. This glimmer of hope for advanced cases signifies the potential of D3 as a complementary therapy.

For prostate cancer patients, the numbers speak volumes. Those with mid-range and high D3 levels enjoyed a 60% and 85% reduction in death risk, respectively, compared to those with low levels. This translates to a 7-fold increase in death risk for those with low D3, highlighting the critical role of D3 in prostate cancer management.

Racial disparities play a role in cancer outcomes. Lower D3 levels in Black Americans may contribute to their higher cancer rates and poorer prognoses. Studies show Black American women and men have, respectively, 25% and 30% higher cancer incidence and 50% higher death rates compared to white Americans. Ensuring adequate D3 levels could be a crucial step towards addressing these disparities.

Remarkably, a single D3 level measured at diagnosis can predict outcomes like metastasis and death in breast cancer patients up to 11 years later. This suggests an exquisite sensitivity of certain cancers to D3 fluctuations, emphasizing the importance of long-term D3 optimization.

Another study looked at the survival rates of women in breast cancer in Norway from 3 separate regions: north middle and south.

Changes in risk of death from breast cancer with season and latitude: From sun exposure and breast cancer survival in Norway

Breast Cancer Res Treat 2007 May;102(3):323-8

This study suggests higher summertime Vitamin D3 levels (due to increased sunlight) may improve breast cancer survival.

Key findings:

- Overall: Summer diagnoses linked to a 15-25% lower risk of death compared to winter diagnoses.

- Younger women (under 50): Those living in southern Norway (more UV exposure) had a 40% lower risk of death than those in the north.

- Older women (over 50): No significant regional difference in survival.

Commentary:

- Actual Vitamin D levels not measured, but assumed deficiency due to Norway's latitude.

- Northern residents consume more fatty fish (dietary Vitamin D source), but still showed worse survival, suggesting sunlight exposure plays a stronger role.

Takeaway: This study provides further evidence linking higher Vitamin D3 levels to improved breast cancer survival, especially in younger women.

(My note, fish also are a source of Vitamin A especially in cod. Vitamin A has been shown to negate the cancer protective effects of Vitamin D3).

The lack of effect in the patients over 50 years of age may be explained by the fact that older people are much less efficient at making Vitamin D3 when exposed to sunlight which highlights the even greater need for supplementation in older age groups.

Similar improvements in survival of breast and lung cancer patients, dependent upon the season of diagnosis have been observed in the UK.

If you want to peruse additional studies and info that reinforce these ideas take a look at the excellent website www.vitamind3world.com

Here is an interesting study found when searching PubMed with the terms

Vitamin D3 AND cancer AND cure

(from 28 total results we find these interesting ones):

Pre-cancerous lesions that often turn into cancer were completely resolved in 2 months with the use of a powerful Vitamin D3 gel.

A novel treatment combination shows promise for porokeratosis:

- Porokeratosis is a skin disorder with atypical patches and an increased risk of skin cancer.

- Existing treatments have limited success.

- This report presents a case of successful treatment with a combined Vitamin D3 analog (calcipotriol) and corticosteroid (betamethasone) gel.

- Significant improvement was seen within 3 weeks, with near-complete resolution in 2 months.

- This appears to be the first documented successful treatment with full resolution using this specific combination.

- The potential effectiveness may be due to the combined action of normalizing keratinocyte growth Vitamin D3 analog (calcipotriol) and reducing inflammation (betamethasone).

- Sun protection and regular monitoring for malignancy remain crucial.

The following treatment includes Vitamin D3 and melatonin (which I also recommend for cancer treatment)

Neuro Endocrinol Lett. 2015;36(8):725-33.

Congenital fibrosarcoma in complete remission with Somatostatin, Bromocriptine, Retinoids, Vitamin D3, Vitamin E, Vitamin C, Melatonin, Calcium, Chondroitin sulfate associated with low doses of Cyclophosphamide in a 14-year Follow up.-

Boy with aggressive leg tumor achieves complete remission with alternative therapy.
- A newborn boy had a large malignant leg tumor (fibrosarcoma).
- Standard treatment (surgery and chemotherapy) was ineffective and risky.
- Parents chose the Di Bella Method, an alternative therapy combining:
  - Somatostatin, Melatonin, Retinoids solubilized in Vit. E, Vit. C, **Vit. D3**, Calcium, and Chondroitin sulfate.
  - Low-dose Cyclophosphamide chemotherapy
- Remarkably, the tumor completely disappeared and remains undetectable after 14 years.
- The boy experienced no significant side effects and enjoys a normal life.

Key points:
- This case study suggests the Di Bella Method may be effective against aggressive cancer.
- Further research is needed to confirm and understand the mechanism of action.

Okay so now here are the real few gems: Cases where high dose Vitamin D3, (50,000 IUs per day), were used in two cases to halt or reverse terminal stage 4 cancer!

The first case was observed by doctors treating 83-year-old women with pancreatic cancer who didn't die after the doctors had given up on her, but 8 months later felt fine and her tumor was shrinking while she was taking 50,000 IUs of D3 per day.

Here is my summary of the full text article:
The Incidental Use of High-Dose Vitamin D3 in Pancreatic Cancer in Case Rep Panceat Cancer. 2016; 2(1): 32–35.

Summary of Pancreatic Cancer and Vitamin D3 Research:
- Pancreatic cancer: Poor prognosis, high mortality rate, limited treatment options.
- Pancreatic cancer is the third most common cause of cancer death in the United States, with more than 40,000 deaths per year. The 5-year survival for all stages of pancreatic adenocarcinoma is ~7.2%.
- Vitamin D3 plays a promising role in cancer prevention and treatment.

Relevant Studies for this Case:

- Higher Vitamin D3 levels may be associated with lower cancer risk, particularly colon cancer.
- In vitro studies suggest Vitamin D3 inhibits pancreatic cancer cell growth and promotes cell death.
- Vitamin D3 receptors (VDRs) regulate key pathways in cancer development and immune response.
- VDRs are abundant in stellate cells, which are part of the stroma of pancreatic cancer.
- The stroma is a supportive tissue that helps the cancer grow and resist treatment by secreting various factors and creating a barrier.
- Activating VDRs can make stellate cells less active and less inflammatory, which may reduce the stroma's harmful effects.
- A study showed that treating pancreatic cancer mice with a vitamin D analogue changed the stellate cells' behavior and gene expression, and improved survival.

Summary of the Case:

- A CT scan performed on February 13, 2015 revealed a 3.6 × 2.7 cm pancreatic tumor in an 83-year-old woman. Most patients with pancreatic tumors of this size or larger usually die within 5.5 months with chemotherapy.

- The patient received one cycle of chemotherapy in March 2015.
- On day 10 of chemo cycle 1, she developed neutropenic fever complicated by atrial fibrillation with rapid ventricular response. She was intubated for a brief time and then recovered to her baseline status. She was discharged on April 19. Based on her frailty, **she was deemed to be a poor candidate for surgery and chemotherapy was not resumed.**
- She started taking high doses of vitamin D3 (50,000 IU /day) and other alternative therapies in April 2015 and continued until December 2015.
- She showed no signs of disease progression or metastasis for 8 months after discharge, despite not receiving any conventional treatment. This is longer than the median progression-free survival of 5.5 months reported in a phase III trial of the chemotherapy regimen she received. Also, a CT scan showed that her tumor had shrunk to CT scan revealed the pancreatic head mass to be 3.1 × 3.0 cm, slightly smaller than previously with a mild increase in

pancreatic duct dilatation. She claimed to be feeling quite well with no difficulty accomplishing her activities of daily living.

- She also had a high vitamin D level over 150 mg/mL and a mild increase in calcium level, which may have contributed to her stable condition.
- The authors acknowledge that there is no causal evidence that vitamin D3 was responsible for this outcome, and that the patient also used other alternative therapies that might have had some effect.
- They suggest that further research is needed to explore the potential benefits of high-dose vitamin D3 for pancreatic cancer patients, especially since it was well tolerated by the patient and did not cause any adverse effects.

Now what follows here is a more anecdotal report reported by a person who is not a medical professional so it is not as reliable as the previous case, but it is very interesting. I doubt someone would go to great lengths to concoct the following story-

You can find this story if you search the internet for- "a tale of two women" ovarian cancer.

You can then find the story at this website link>
https://pandemicsurvivor.com/2009/06/28/a-tale-of-
two-women/

A Tale of Two Women – Ovarian cancer

In February of 2008 we got some bad news. Our
friend's daughter had cancer. This was very
devastating to us because we had two daughters, so
we knew how much our friends were hurting. She
was only 19 years old and the threat of cancer
hanging over her was certainly frightening. She was
a heady smart intelligent young woman who loved
to spend time reading and working on her
computer. **She did not spend a lot of time outside
and she had the loveliest white complexion that a
lot of people would say was most pleasing**.

We told our friends about the Vitamin D thing and
how it could help prevent and maybe even help the
healing process. Vitamin D3, it seems works, along
several pathways to help heal disease. Number one
it helps at a genetic level to tell immature tumor
cells that they are just that and to stop growing or
undergo cellular apoptosis. The D3 also helps the
blood supply network that is feeding the tumor to
stop growing from a genetic level because this is
not the normal design of the body or angiogenesis.
Also, it raises the level of innate immunity, so the
body develops appropriate defenses such as
cathelicidin antimicrobial peptides, phagocytes, and

neutrophil granulocytes that help destroy and absorb 'bad cells' and 'foreign bodies' in the blood system. There is also an aid to T-cell regulation in this complex system of immunity. And if you are taking chemo one of the problems is thrombosis and Vitamin D3 helps to control this issue as well.

It would seem that if any of this were true that you would want to get your serum level of 25(OH)D up to that of a sunny country or about 54 ng/ml to 90 ng/ml to allow the body to heal itself. However, our friends, one of them a medical professional, thought that if there was anything to this understanding of Vitamin D that the cancer 'experts' or oncologist would have long ago begun this practice of maintaining a 'sunny country' level of Vitamin D3 in cancer patients. This seemed like a reasonable decision at the time. I just can't imagine the advice and what type that you would get if a family member had cancer.

The treatment protocols for our friend seemed to progress well through the year and they thought that with the combination of radiation and chemo that they had the cancer under control. On the Friday before thanksgiving they decided to take their daughter back to the hospital for evaluation because she was having a lot of problems with headaches. It turns out that she had more tumors that had come back, so they decided to begin treatment again on the following Monday. Their daughter died on

Saturday before they had a chance to begin treatment. We are grieving.

In February of 2008 we got some more bad news. My brother called to say that he had a girlfriend that was in a serious way with cancer. It turns out that she had ovarian cancer that was discovered two years prior. She had surgery and had the tumors removed as well as her uterus. She was told at the time that the cancer had metastasized to so many places in her body that she would have only two years to live. She had a great job in New York City but decided that life should be lived to its fullest and she would come back home and take a walk on the wild side. Who could blame her for this action?

My brother said that she had internal bleeding as she was passing blood and that all of her lymph nodes were swollen all over her body and that she had other lumps. It seems that her medical insurance had expired and that she 'had enough' of the medical system. With not any energy left she decided to just go to bed to die. My brother wanted to help but did not know what to do. He called to ask if there was anything to this Vitamin D. I told him that I did not think that it would help anyone who was this far along with developed cancer and that the best thing he could do was to call the woman's oncologist expert that we have in our family to see if he had any suggestions and to get this woman to a doctor.

My brother decided that he would just tell her about the Vitamin D and see what she wanted to do. She agreed that if it could even give her any relief that she was willing to try it. **She decided to take 50,000 IU of D3 per day or 1.25 milligrams for three months**. She took other supplements as well like calcium, Vitamin A from fish liver oil, chelated magnesium, zinc, Vitamin C, and a Vitamin B complex. I told my brother that it sounded like the alphabet of nutrition. She had also read that it would help balance the body's system to drink bicarbonate of soda every day, so she did that. In late October I got a call from the woman. She wanted to call to say thank you for helping them find out about the information on Vitamin D3. **She said that all of her symptoms were gone and that she had the most energy that she had in twenty-five years**. She was out looking for work. I asked her about the Vitamin D3 and how she had taken it and **she said that she took a 50,000 IU per day until the bottle was gone or 100 days** (at this level of use you could expect toxicity to begin at about six months or more) and then took a 50,000 IU once per week. After she realized that she was not going to die she went to a doctor that advised her to keep taking the Vitamin D3 at one 50,000IU per week as it would certainly do no harm.

I just did not know what to think at this point. Had my brother exaggerated the symptoms of her cancer? Was there some kind of spontaneous remission of the cancer? She had reunited with her mother and they had the church praying for her so maybe it was a miracle of God and whatever the path it certainly is a miracle of God. Anyway, I could not wrap my mind around this. Maybe the researchers are correct but just did not know how correct they are. I understand that there are ongoing trials for the prevention of cancer with Vitamin D3 but has anyone thought about trials for the treatment of cancer. Are we so tied into a system that only responds to profit that we cannot just help heal people and consider their health a profit?

I checked just a couple of weeks ago and my brother said, 'yeah she is doing just fine'. I still do not know what to think!?

If you think you have any symptoms of cancer go to a doctor! You may also want to think about using D3 to get your serum level to that of sunny country as it will not do any harm and may help you significantly. Also, please consider you diet to determine if you are getting the correct foods for essential nutrition.

Here are some more cancer related Vitamin D3 stories that appear on the high dose Vitamin D3 search engine at my website JeffTbowles.com when you search the term cancer:

Lytbender
Varicose veins
October 16, 2012 at 8:03 pm
hey Above2
I have been taken 50,000 units of D3 with K2 daily for 8 months now and have never felt better. As you noted I sleep like a baby, lost weight, have not been sick except for a urticaria skin condition when I am stressed from air travel. I think the D3 is helping that too. I am a vegan and had not been getting enough D3, K2 and Vitamin A. **My blood levels are at 150**. I am amazed how this has helped me. My varicose veins are almost gone, my gums no longer bleed, **my skin cancers are gone.** I could go on and on. I first read Jeff Bowles book on high dose Vit D3 to start me on it. I think this is the missing link to our health.

I am 74 years old and a retired mechanic. In my forties I started getting all kinds of lesions on my forearms: discolorations, growths, liver spots, bumps, etc. Some of the lesions had different color spots on them, as in precancerous lesions. Thinking that this was caused by the chemicals I was using at work I started keeping my sleeves buttoned down while working. After the increased D3 (summer 2017) the lesions started to kind of dry up, get crusty. You could scrape them with a fingernail, and they would come off like dead skin after a sun burn. Some would show a little blood and then scab over. When the scab fell off there was a small pink patch where the lesion had been. Eventually the pink patch became the same color as the surrounding skin. My arms still have some marks, but I am no longer reluctant to wear short sleeve shirts in public. I just cannot believe the transformation. I can look at my forearms now. <u>This book will change your life forever.</u>

By A Haddonon 27 September 2015

I read this book while on holiday in July 2015. This book has changed my life for good. We went on a cruise, mainly because I was unable to walk due to my condition fibromyalgia and chronic fatigue syndrome. Jeff Bowles writes about high doses of Vitamin D3. I'm a very pale skinned Welsh lady who never ever goes in the sun unless I'm protected. As soon as I got home, I order the D3 supplement along with K2 as stated in the book. Within 3 days I was able to put my feet on the floor without the pain, within one month I was able to get out of bed unaided and also clean my home without help. Since July I have bought a bike and I ride 13km daily, I walk my dogs 3km daily and I have been discharged from hospital. I have also lost 18lbs in weight. I'm 45 and I'm getting around like I did in my teens**. My mum had cancer and was wasting away. You should see her now.** I've also started my dogs and friends' dogs on it and it's cured my friend's dog of arthritis and my spaniel is now running like a pup. What an amazing book and a big thank you from a little village in Wales to Mr. Jeff Bowles.

And finally I heard from a Dr. Tim Ioannides who is a Florida dermatologist who invented a treatment for untreatable skin cancer using HPV vaccine that completely cured a 97+year old women of a large number of inoperable skin cancers on her legs (squamous cell) by injecting them with HPV vaccine after he had pre-treated her 6 weeks earlier with the vaccine. The immune system just ate them up. He told me he got the idea after reading my first Vitamin D3 book where I boasted that using PubMed, anyone can find a cure for any disease in 30 minutes to 30 days just by reading all the pub med studies concerning that disease and putting the facts (pieces) to together like a puzzle. He tried it and this was how he found his skin cancer cure. Here is a link to the news report on his discovery. He had to enlist the help of a senior female doctor at the hospital because he was not a full-time staff member. The report implies it was her idea, but it was all Tim's-

Doctors recognized for treating 97-year-old woman's squamous cell cancer with HPV vaccine

Janet Begley, Special to TCPALM

243

(this illustration omitted in paperback-please see the eBook or email Bannedcovidbook@gmail.com for the pdf)

A Port St. Lucie dermatologist was recognized for his approach in treating a 97-year-old woman's squamous cell skin cancer tumors with the human papillomavirus.

PORT ST. LUCIE — A Treasure Coast dermatologist has been recognized by the Journal of the American Medical Association for his treatment of squamous cell cancer with the human papillomavirus vaccine Gardasil 9.

Dr. Tim Ioannides, from Treasure Coast Dermatology in Port St. Lucie; along with Dr. Anna Nichols, a dermatologist and an assistant professor in the Dr. Phillip Frost Department of Dermatology and Cutaneous Surgery at the University of Miami Comprehensive Cancer Center, published a study in 2018 in which a 97-year-old woman's squamous cell skin cancer tumors disappeared after she was injected with the HPV vaccine.

The patient recently celebrated her 100th birthday without a relapse.

Here is a link to a video about the discovery>>
http://med.miami.edu/news/sylvesters-use-of-hpv-vaccine-to-treat-patient-with-skin-tumors-reported-in

Well, Dr Tim also mentioned to me that he had a male cancer patient who had terminal cancer but was cured by taking high doses of Vitamin D3. He then noted that the patient stopped taking the high dose D3 and the cancer came back. I pressed him for more details, but he is being tight lipped about it as I think he is trying to apply for some sort of use-patent. I will ask him to give me an update and add it here later if it is forthcoming.

So that'd about it. If I was diagnosed with cancer, I would immediately start taking at least 50,000 IU of D3 per day and I recommend this to anyone else. There will be no Big Pharma study on high dose D3 for cancer as it is not patentable, and they cannot make any money from it.

Even if Vitamin D3 + cofactors are the best treatment for all cancers, you will never hear about it from the vast majority of doctors and never from Big pharma for a long, long, time. In fact, I expect there will be a major active campaign to discredit and outlaw Vitamin D3 before long by those who have a financial interest in the cancer and illness industry.

I propose that we the guinea pig population of the US for Big Pharma and modern medicine take it upon ourselves to do a large experiment of taking high dose Vitamin D3 for every case of cancer that ever arises, and report back to me with your results good or bad. You can take it along with your conventional therapy. You can share your experiences with me at my email address at: jeffbo at aol dot com. I will add all your results to the high dose Vitamin D3 1,000+ case studies search engine.

But the good news is that you if you take the information to heart in this book and start a Vitamin D3+cofactors regimen, you will very likely never ever get cancer, so I likely will never hear from you. So, if you want to help you can convince anyone you know who gets cancer to give high dose Vitamin D3 a try.

Appendix A - The Big Vitamin D3 Mistake

Dimitrios T. Papadimitriou

See e-book or request pdf from
BannedCovidBook@gmail.com (omitted for
brevity)

link> https://www.amazon.com/dp/B07ZBP8QZZ

Appendix B: The Human Hibernation Syndrome-

In my best-selling book:

The Miraculous Results of Extremely High Doses of The Sunshine Hormone Vitamin D3 My Experiment with Huge Doses of D3 From 25,000 To 50,000 To 100,000 IUs A Day Over A 1 Year Period,

I asked why would evolution create such a hormone that decreases in the winter months and gives you a whole host of diseases and chronic problems? This should not exist. Evolution should have eliminated this problem long ago by killing off those who were vulnerable to Vitamin D3 deficiency diseases in short order then the problem would not exist after that, but it persists with a vengeance!

I wondered if there might be some sort of important evolutionary purpose to the fact that evolution wants us to be sick in the winter months. That is when I came up with the idea of the Human Hibernation Syndrome.

You just have to imagine what it might have been like in the distant past when dark skinned humans started migrating north into climates of weaker sun. Eventually some of these humans would migrate so far north that they would have to endure cold, snowy, dark winters. Many animals from bears to squirrels and even perennial plants like trees show us the best way to survive extremely cold, and likely famine-plagued winters is to HIBERNATE. Shut down energy-wasting system to as low a level as possible, and just hunker down and try to wait out the months of famine and freezing.

However, before you hibernate, evolution would want you to fatten up as much as possible before winter set in, and that is exactly what brown bears do. When their Vitamin D3 levels drop by about 70% in the early fall it triggers an insatiable sense of hunger that causes female bears to increase their body weight by 70% or more! They go on an eating rampage dictated by low Vitamin D3 levels. I believe a similar thing happens in humans.

Evolution seems to have perfected hibernation in the bear, but it seems like it still is trying to find the best solution for humans. So instead of just a straight up- "go to your cave and sleep for 4 months", hibernation in humans seems to be approaching this outcome but hasn't made it there yet. Vitamin D3 deficiency can make you depressed so you don't want to leave your cave or abode. It can give you extreme fatigue like chronic fatigue syndrome It can also give you temporarily chronic diseases like MS, arthritis, asthma, ulcerative colitis, even the flu etc. to further reduce your interest in leaving the shelter and wasting precious energy wandering around in the snow during a time of little to no food. Evolution basically tries to cripple you, so you ride out the winter famine. This protects you from starving to death by burning up too many of your precious calories.

Evolution also likely caused your body to conserve critical resources and not waste them doing repair and remodeling of injuries and defective cells and tissues while in starvation mode. This can be seen in a rat experiment where they broke the legs of rats and let the bones heal with and without Vitamin D3 supplementation. The D3 deficient rats had shoddy repairs where it looked like there was a glob of clay pressed around the area where the bone was broken. In the D3 supplemented rats, the break completely healed, much stronger than in the controls, with no trace of the break's existence! This also may explain why Vitamin D3 deficient individuals can accumulate bone spurs, injuries, and cysts that never heal, and even why some D3 deficient immune systems might just let cancer cells linger in the body rather than killing them off. Maybe defective tissues and cells can be used as future sources of nourishment to ward off starvation.

Evolution even prepares your body to survive near freezing conditions by boosting your blood sugar (diabetes) which acts like ethylene glycol anti-freeze in a car, and salt levels, like the salt we use to keep the streets free of ice. Evolution also raises

250

your blood pressure which allows more gases to dissolve in your blood which dramatically lowers its freezing temperature. People with high blood pressure tend to crave salt.

Back in ancient times, this human hibernation condition might last for three to four months but quickly would be reversed when the stronger spring sun melted the snow, allowing humans to go back out into nature and boost their Vitamin D3 levels by exposing their skin to sunlight.

However, since the 1980's, most of us have been taking the advice of the medical community to stay out of the sun and use sunscreen whenever we go outside! This has led to a situation where, I believe, most modern-day humans suffer from a permanent case of the Human Hibernation Syndrome (HHS). This is evidenced by the explosive rise of almost all diseases known to man since the 1980's! Cancer, asthma, autism, asthma, obesity, you name it, there has been a huge epidemic of it starting around 1980. These epidemics can only be corrected by abandoning doctors' advice and going out and getting suntanned every summer or taking Vitamin D3 supplements at much higher doses than recommended by current guidelines.

Appendix C: Some Fun Speculation-

Which Came First the Disease of Cancer? Or the Tropic of Cancer?

See e-book or request pdf from BannedCovidbook@gmail.com (omitted for brevity)

link> https://www.amazon.com/dp/B07ZBP8QZZ

Appendix D: Diseases Caused by Vitamin D3 Deficiency- Excerpt From my Book (With Notes):

The Miraculous Results of Extremely High Doses of The Sunshine Hormone Vitamin D3 My Experiment with Huge Doses of D3 From 25,000 To 50,000 To 100,000 Iu A Day Over A 1 Year Period

From My Book about high dose Vitamin D3 (with notes)-

See e-book or request pdf (omitted for brevity)

link> https://www.amazon.com/dp/B07ZBP8QZZ

Appendix E Some Additional Interesting Abstracts Concerning Magnesium:

See e-book or request pdf (omitted for brevity)

link> https://www.amazon.com/dp/B07ZBP8QZZ

Appendix F Side Effects of High Strength (Active) Vitamin D: Calcitriol

(Calcitriol is formed when Vitamin D3 (cholecalciferol) is activated in the kidney, but doctors can prescribe the active form under special circumstances).

- bone pain,
- changes in behavior
- constipation
- diarrhea
- drowsiness
- dry mouth
- eye pain
- eye redness,
- eye sensitivity to light
- headache
- heart rate abnormalities
- increased thirst
- loss of appetite
- metallic taste in the mouth
- muscle pain
- muscle weakness
- nausea,
- photophobia (night blindness)
- severe pain in the upper stomach spreading to the back.
- slow growth (in a child taking calcitriol)
- stomach pain
- urination-excessive

- vomiting
- weakness
- weight loss

It is an interesting and instructive exercise to compare these side effects of activated Vitamin D3 to the various deficiency symptoms of its cofactors (especially magnesium!).

Appendix G: Symptoms and Causes of low Potassium Low Potassium

See e-book request pdf from Bannedcovidbook@gmail.com (omitted for brevity)

link> https://www.amazon.com/dp/B07ZBP8QZZ

Appendix H: An Example of a Serious Disease Caused by Soils Depleted of the Mineral Selenium

Occurrence of Diseases Caused by Selenium Deficiency (Geographic Distribution of Keshan disease exactly corresponds to the Map Pattern of Selenium Deficient Soil in China)

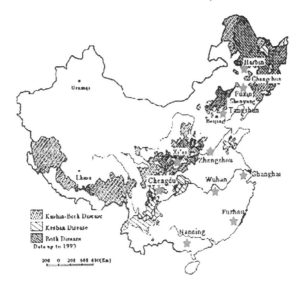

Incidence of Keshan Disease Vs. Selenium Deficient Soil- An Exact Match

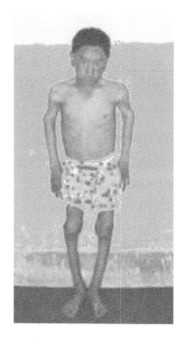

Keshan Disease Patient-
Muscular Dystrophy, Loss of Appetite, Nausea

The bottom-line lesson of this appendix G is to make you aware of how dangerous long-term mineral deficiencies caused by depleted soils can be! This one is easy to see. Magnesium, zinc, boron deficiencies disease can be more subtle and harder to see, but just as dangerous!

Appendix I- A Quick Review of Studies Beginning in the 1920's through 1947 concerning Vitamin D in PubMed-Titles Only

See e-book or request pdf (omitted for brevity)

link> https://www.amazon.com/dp/B07ZBP8QZZ

Made in the USA
Las Vegas, NV
14 October 2024